Your Heart

May Be A

Ticking Time Bomb!

How to Save Your Own Life
BEFORE the Bomb Squad Comes
with Drugs, Stents, and Surgery

DR. DAN PILGREEN

LOS ANGELES, CA

Your Heart May Be A Ticking Time Bomb!

Published by Solutions Press, Newport Beach, CA

Every effort has been made to make this book as complete and as accurate as possible, but no warranty or fitness is implied. The information provided is on an "as is" basis. The advice and strategies contained herein may not be suitable for every situation. The author and the publisher shall have neither liability nor responsibility to any person or entity with respect to any loss or damages arising from the information contained in this book.

ISBN: 978-0-9827646-5-7

Printed in the United States of America

First Printing: May 2011

Disclaimer

The information in this book is for informational purposes only. It is general information and not intended to be used in any way to diagnose, treat, cure, or prevent any disease. The sole purpose is to highlight and present nutritional information and offer protocols and suggestions for nutritional maintenance and support overall health.

You should never use the information in this book without consulting your own physician or to replace conventional medical care. It is the sole responsibility of the user to determine if any recommendations in this book are appropriate. The author is not responsible for the information in this book or any inadvertent omissions or errors

Never postpone or delay proper medical treatment. Always seek immediate and prompt care from a licensed medical professional. Do not start a diet, exercise, or nutritional program without contacting your personal physician.

What doctors say...

"This is cutting edge information. If you want to know what to take and why with all the supporting documentation, this book is a must read. Not only do I recommend this program to my patients, I follow it myself and I put my mother on it. If you want to know what the best vitamins, exercise and diet is just ask what doctors recommend for their own families."

— Dr. Gelda Adarme, M.D.

"Your Heart May Be A Ticking Time Bomb is a wonderful and refreshing look into the one of the most important, yet overlooked, health issues affecting the global population in general. Dr. Pilgreen has been blessed with a candid courage, an extensive knowledge, a passionate heart, and a determined mind to assemble and present very comprehensive, yet easy to read and apply, material for all to enjoy. It is not only highly recommended, but it is a must read for all, without exception."

— Dr. Ara Yaghjian, D.C.

"The chapters on amino acids are excellent and the concept of synergism really makes this program stand out. If you want to get rid of your drugs start this natural program now."

— Dr. Travis Huteson, D.C.

"You only know if you get results and they have been spectacular. Many of the recommendations are simple to follow and the exercise program is very effective at lowering blood pressure. Much needed updates of all the research on each nutrient makes you know why you need to take each nutrient. The new research on each vitamin is eye opening and encouraging. I like that it's not only a complete but effective program. This book is a must read."

— Dr. Richard Bulbuk, D.C.

Dedication

I would like to thank my wife, Beate, for her love and support. I am also grateful for my two children, Claire and Noah, who inspired me to write this book so I would be there for them and not end up a statistic like so many others.

Special to thanks to Dr. Michael Bradley, my brother and inspiration until his passing; Linus Pauling, who inspired me early on with his lecture series on vitamin C; Dr. Mike Cessna, visionary teacher of alternative health care; Dr. Rolla Pennel, one of the greatest minds of the 20th century on natural treatment.

Proverbs 15:7b: "The lips of the wise spread knowledge."

What patients say...

"I have congestive heart failure and could only walk a few blocks; today I walked over five miles. I sleep better. I have a new lease on life."

— Ben Morris, Moreno Valley, CA

"Since I have started the supplements my sugar levels have gone down and my A1C test dropped a full point. If I stop the supplements my blood sugar goes up 10 to 15 points."

— Debra Lovelace, Florida

"I feel like a kid again. I have more energy and I only need one pill at night as my blood sugar has dropped from 134 to 101. My medical doctor recommended Dr. Pilgreen's program."

— Jeanette Bond, Los Angeles, CA

"My father-in-law Alex Kovach has so many health problems, it's hard to keep track. He has heart problems and diabetes along with macular degeneration. The drug they gave him caused an autoimmune disorder. We started the supplements and now he can sleep for the first time in two years."

— Lisa Chan & Alex Kovach, Granite City, IL

"My whole family is on this program as we have a history of heart disease and high blood pressure."

— Deanne Smith, Los Angeles, CA

"My blood sugar has returned to normal for the first time in six months after starting the program."

— Jose Pelayos, Los Angeles, CA

What patients say...

"I followed Dr. Pilgreen's program and it returned my blood pressure to normal."

— Nash Powle, Arcadia, CA

"I have had heart trouble for the last ten years. Three years ago I had bypass surgery and that was one terrible experience. I was still not my old self two years after the surgery. I had absolutely no energy. I was always on the go prior to the operation and now I could barely walk my dog. I started vitamins, exercise and diet. In one month I was back to my old self. My doctor even stopped my diabetes medication because I had improved so much."

— Martha Lewis, Las Vegas, NV

"My blood pressure has dropped from 170/90 to 150/80 in one month on this regimen. I really feel the difference. I have more energy now."

— Kathleen DeCardenas, Bell, CA

"My doctors have treated me for the last ten years for heart problems. I take over five medications. I really didn't feel better and I didn't like the side effects of the drugs. I have been on the vitamins and diet for 12 months. I have been able to stop most of my medications and I can do a lot of things I had given up on."

— Hans Venohr, Crailsheim, Germany

"I have tried just about everything on the market for my health and my heart condition. They did not work. Once I started taking the nutrients everything was better. I walked up a hill today that I would have never been able to climb before this. Truly amazing.

— Ed Mallon, Rosemead, CA

What patients say...

"Richard has had quadruple bypass surgery and has congestive heart failure and diabetes. Since taking the supplements he has more energy, looks better, his color is back. The nurses at the cardiac rehab unit can't believe how much better he is. He used to be on oxygen but he rarely needs it now. Thanks so much."

— Sharon and Richard Moody, Tustin, CA

"I have suffered from chronic infections for years. I've taken numerous courses of antibiotic therapy with no results. I always have mucus and phlegm in my lungs. I have been to too many doctors with no relief. Since taking the supplements I have experienced more energy. I have a smaller amount of phlegm and not as much mucus as before."

— David Gehl, Los Angeles, CA

"I had bypass surgery which left me with no strength and I started getting panic attacks and nightmares. It was so bad that I didn't want to leave the house. I barely made it to the mailbox. I didn't think the program would help. Well let me tell you it's been a miracle. I'm out of the house with more energy and going to a dance camp. My anxiety is gone, no more nightmares and my strength has returned."

— Dennis Boxell, Sunland, CA

"I'm 45 years old. I had very bad chest pains and went to the hospital. Doctors told me I had a heart attack. They did an angiogram and said I had a blocked artery. I did not want bypass surgery. By a miracle a doctor recommended the supplements. After six months I feel great, walk two miles a day, and have no chest pain."

— Fuad Hamati, Los Angeles, CA

Contents

Your Heart May Be A Ticking Time Bomb!

Preface

Who needs to read this book? Everyone who is:
- Concerned about preventing or treating heart disease.
- Seeking a nutritional alternative to conventional heart disease treatment.

Why? Because the question is not *whether* you will get heart disease; it is *when* you will.

The primary goal of this book is to educate you about heart disease and its prevention, the nutrients needed by your body, nutrient depletion caused by inadequate diet and pharmaceutical drugs, and what nutrients to take, the best diet and most effective exercise regimen.

Happy, heart-healthy reading.

Dr. Dan Pilgreen, D.C.

What patients say...

"I was taking medications for my diabetes, angina (chest pains), and high blood pressure. I'm so pleased with this program. The results are fantastic. I can't thank you enough."

— Gloria B. Flores, Carson , CA

"My husband has high blood pressure (around 180). We have weaned him off of his medication, his blood pressure dropped 30 to 40 points. He has more energy. This program is amazing."

— Connie and Walter Sakawaye, Los Angeles, CA

"I had had two stents and didn't want to do that again. After this program my doctor checked me and said my blood flow was perfect after a thallium stress test."

— Ralph Beacker, Lakewood, CA

"I have heart problems. I have more energy since starting the supplements. I can walk around the block, which I couldn't do before. I'm sleeping better."

— Linea Davis, Pasadena, CA

1

About Heart Disease

*"Half the costs of illness are wasted on
conditions that could be prevented."*

*— Dr. Joseph Pizzorno
Author, "Total Wellness"*

I wasn't prepared for the phone call. The voice on the other end of the line was urgent. "Your father has had a heart attack." Those seven words pierce the hearts of thousands of people every day just as they did mine.

At the time, I had just started practice as an associate doctor. At the age of 24, I was one of the youngest graduates of chiropractic medical school in California. When I put down the phone, I turned to my boss, Dr. Smith, a large bear of a man. I wrapped my arms around his huge frame and cried. He told me, "Go be with your father."

The doctor who operated on my dad said he had so much plaque in his arteries that his aorta simply shut down. The doctor tried to clean out the blockage but could only get the catheters down to mid thigh. My dad's arteries were like old, stopped up rusty pipes.

Intermittent claudication. It's the reason Dad had to sell his restaurant. The arteries in his legs were so clogged that he could barely make it to the end of the lunch counter before burning pain stopped him in his tracks. Whenever we went somewhere, he would always wind up saying, "Go ahead, I'll catch up."

That horrible day my dad said he hadn't been feeling well. On his way to the VA hospital he had the heart attack. Two days later, he died.

I had thought that I would be okay with it as he was in his late seventies, but the pain was completely overwhelming and nearly unbearable. I felt helpless and angry.

What happened to my dad could happen to you or one of your loved ones. Dad's heart was a ticking time bomb. It was ticking down to the final detonation. Tick, tick, tick...

The facts about heart attack and heart disease

Medical technology was not as advanced then as it is now, but it probably would not have helped my dad anyway. Even today, with new advances in medicine, people drop dead of heart attacks—also called coronary thrombosis and myocardial infarction—like flies.

To avoid my pain, I began to fill my time researching and studying heart disease. Here's some of what I found:

- Every 33 seconds, someone dies of a heart attack in the United States—a total death count equivalent to five fully loaded jumbo jets crashing every day.
- Heart attacks are the number one killer followed by cancer, stroke, and diabetes.
- Two thirds of all deaths are attributable to heart disease and related conditions.
- Seventy percent of all fatal heart attacks are sudden and without warning.

Over 700,000 Americans will have a new heart attack and 500,000 will have a recurrent attack every year. Not only is the number of attacks increasing, but people who are under medical care have a 70 percent chance of having a second heart attack. Here are some more figures to chew on. In 2006:

- Coronary bypass operations: 1,285,000
- Angioplasties: 427,000
- Diagnostic catheterizations (angiograms): 1,471,000

That's a lot of procedures. Coronary heart disease (CHD) comprises more than half of all cardiovascular events in men and women under age 75. The lifetime risk of developing CHD after the age of 40 is 49 percent for men and 32 percent for women. Alarming? You bet. This is a call for all baby boomers to carefully consider being proactive to prevent heart disease.

The cost of heart disease is staggering. The heart disease business is booming. The American Heart Association's latest statistics showed that $151.6 billion was spent on heart disease in 2007.

Shocking headlines

Unfortunately heart attack headlines abound:

- Major League Umpire Dies of a Heart Attack
- Assistant Head Soccer Coach Dead at 51 of Heart Attack
- News Anchor Dies: Heart Attack Suspected
- President Clinton to Have Quadruple Bypass Surgery

Fans watched in horror as John McSherry staggered around home plate and collapsed during the opening game of the 1996 major league baseball season. He was later pronounced dead of a massive heart attack. The 6'2" McSherry was officially listed at 328 pounds, but some say he was closer to 400 pounds.

In 2007, Glenn Myernick, an assistant coach for the U.S. soccer team, died suddenly after suffering a heart attack at 51. Myernick, however, was in good shape and was not overweight.

And, everyone was stunned when noted NBC news anchor Tim Russert died of a heart attack in 2009. Russert's doctor, Dr. Michael A. Newman, said in an interview, "Mr. Russert had coronary artery disease, but no symptoms. He had done everything he was supposed to do to manage the disease; Mr. Russert was managing his risk factors well through diet and exercise."

Research has shown that heart disease begins in our 20's. Autopsies on auto casualties and Korean and Vietnam War soldiers in their 20's showed heart disease in coronary arteries. If you are over 40, you have a 39 percent chance of dying from a heart attack.

With such a heart attack epidemic occurring, was Tim Russert doing all that he could? Are there things that he could have done to prevent a heart attack other than diet and exercise?

In 2004, even with the best medical care in the world, President Bill Clinton had to have quadruple bypass surgery. There were no warning signs. The doctors completely missed his heart disease. Six years later, he was back in the news. He had stents put in because the initial bypass treatment was not designed to reverse heart disease, only to treat the symptoms. His doctor said Clinton had done everything right since his bypass—eating well, exercising, and controlling his blood pressure and cholesterol levels.

But here's the thing: President Clinton didn't have a stent deficiency; he had damage to his arteries due to oxidation. Lack of numerous vitamins and minerals started the artery damage in the first place.

Heart attacks overlooked in women

Women are just as vulnerable to heart attacks as men. Heart disease, once thought the sole domain of men, is now just as common in women after menopause. In fact, one out of every three women will die of a heart attack.[1]

The preconceived bias that women don't have heart attacks has led to many women being sent home from emergency rooms with dangerously false diagnoses of heartburn or muscle pain. Some suffer permanent heart damage and even death due to these misdiagnoses. This notion is now changing due to the increased incidence of heart attacks in women. But even if a doctor is sharp enough to catch a woman's heart attack, she could still wind up with a bypass operation and a lifetime sentence to drugs.

Heart attacks and modern medicine

Most people think modern medicine has a handle on the heart attack epidemic, but the facts speak for themselves. Along with heart attacks, there are epidemics of high blood pressure, elevated cholesterol levels, heart palpitations, chest pain, and irregular heartbeat (arrhythmias).

In over 40 years, treatment hasn't changed nor has modern medicine been able to find a cure. New drugs, new surgical procedures, new technology—all have the same old result.

There have been some successes with cholesterol lowering drugs, but only with people who already have advanced heart disease. These drugs are totally ineffective, however, for men over 65 and for all women.

I am not bashing medical practitioners; they are highly skilled and caring professionals who possess the best minds in the country. I *am* bashing the basic assumption that drugs or surgery can solve everything *without looking at the underlying cause.*

The good news is, there are things you can do and vitamins and nutrients you can take to stop heart disease, prevent it, or even reverse it, but you need to educate yourself about them. That's why, I hope, you are reading this book.

What's the cause of heart disease?

Modern medicine says that faulty nutrition is not the cause of heart disease. Really? You would be surprised to know that a recent study determined that eighty percent of all medical doctors take vitamin E to protect against heart disease yet don't recommend it to their patients. Unfortunately, there is still peer pressure in the medical profession—no one wants to be known as the "vitamin nut."

Modern medicine says that cholesterol is the problem. Half of all heart attacks, however, occur in people with normal cholesterol levels.

Another quarter of all people who have heart attacks have no risk factors whatsoever. That means they didn't smoke or drink, they weren't obese, they exercised regularly, their cholesterol levels were normal, and some were vegetarians. Many were doing everything that their doctors told them—just like Tim Russert—and they died anyway.

When you have a heart attack you are sent to get an array of outrageously expensive tests that indicate abnormalities. Then they'll rush you in for a bypass or stent and, most assuredly, you will get at least four to six drug prescriptions for your trouble. None of these procedures, though, reverses the disease, they only to treat the symptoms.

Nutrient deficiency: the silent killer

Long-term drug use, by the way, causes vitamin deficiencies. Vast amounts of scientific research prove that the lack of proper vitamin C, and many other nutrients, causes heart disease. A deficiency in vitamin C results in sub clinical scurvy, which is one of the main causes of heart disease. "Sub clinical" means that you do not get the symptoms of scurvy, but you get the damage to the vascular system that eventually injures the artery wall.

Here's what happens when your body lacks vitamin C:

- Inflammation starts in the vessel wall where the muscle cells are and causes cracks in the wall.
- The body sends white blood cells to engulf the inflamed cells.
- This causes debris that turns into a foamy mess.
- The body covers the messy goop and tries to patch it, which causes bumps.
- Cholesterol accumulates on the sticky bumps forming a fibrous cap that pushes into the artery, making them larger.
- The fibrous cap can break off and cause a heart attack or clot (when the fast moving blood hits the plaque).

So it's not the cholesterol that causes the problem; it simply sticks to the injured artery.

When adequate amounts of vitamin C, amino acids, lysine and proline, and the mineral copper are present in sufficient quantities, blood vessel cracks do not occur.

Without cracks, there are no lipoprotein-a patches and no collection of cholesterol. Thus, there are no heart attacks due to blocking of the artery and the death of the heart muscle.

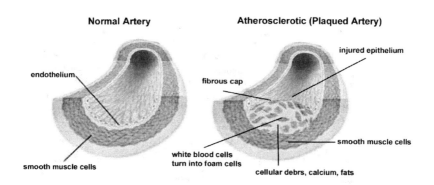

The worst part about chronic low-grade vitamin C deficiency is that it is a silent killer. You cannot feel vitamin deficiencies. Of the more than one million heart attacks a year, 250,000 are sudden and fatal. That means one quarter of heart attack victims die without any warning signs.

In addition to vitamin C's major role in preventing heart disease, research shows that many vitamins, amino acids, and minerals also play a critical part in preventing blood vessel damage and ensuing heart disease.

I talk more about drugs and nutrient deficiency in Chapter 4.

Back to my story

As I said previously, the end of my dad's life was the beginning of my exploration of heart disease and heart attack prevention. My research began to point me in the direction of natural therapeutics, because it was clear that drugs were not fixing the problem and there was a need for natural treatments without the frequent debilitating side effects of conventional medicine.

I had been in practice for 23 years and had treated over 10,000 patients. I saw heart disease, high cholesterol, and high blood pressure at epidemic proportions, as well as diabetes and stroke. So I widened my research and began delving into research about vitamins and illness prevention in general.

One of the most striking research articles I found was from the *Journal of the American Medical Association*. It reported a **40 percent decrease in all cancers** when a simple 200-microgram dose of selenium was administered to a study group. Wow!

Quality of research is key

The studies that I cite throughout this book all were double blind, controlled studies performed at major institutions with thousands of participants. That makes them very credible to me.

When someone says to me that there is some new nutrient that will cure everything from flat feet to dandruff to cancer, I'm always skeptical. That doesn't mean that it couldn't be true in the future, but if the research doesn't support the claims, I have hard time believing it.

Likewise, products hawked on the radio or TV such as betaglucan, collustrum, alpha lipoic acid, mangosteen, and Acai berry are not the wonder cures they are touted to be. Solid, quality research doesn't currently exist for these substances.

I've always told my patients that if it's good today, it will be good in six months or a year from now. Until the research seems promising, it seems prudent and rational to wait.

Most holistic health marketing produces fear and the need for the product right away. After 23 years of practice using vitamins and minerals on real patients, I can tell you that hype didn't produce the results.

The same fear tactics, by the way, are used with great success by drug companies who trumpet marginal success and downplay the side effects and lack of benefits.

Greed treats the symptoms but doesn't cure the problem

If vitamins and minerals, amino acids and various neutirceuticals are so good why isn't this research on the front page of every newspaper? Why doesn't the media pound away at the phenomenal strides in nutrition research? The reason is simple: greed. Much of the media is backed by large pharmaceutical companies that have no interest in public health, other than to make huge profits on marginally effective treatments and to suppress viable alternatives.

While studies show that nutrient therapy works as well as a bypass, angioplasty, or drug therapy, the heart disease medication business alone is a $200 billion a year industry. By treating the symptoms rather than curing the problem, drug companies create lifetime patients. The underlying nutrient deficiency that causes heart disease in the first place is never addressed under the current medical model, which seeks to make money by treating symptoms only.

2

Conventional Medical Treatment

"The doctor of the future will give no medicine, but will interest his patients in the care of the human frame, in diet, and in the cause and prevention of disease."

— Thomas Alva Edison

Before I get into natural alternatives, I want to look deeper into standard or conventional medical treatment and discuss what current research says about its effectiveness. Does it really work and can you do more? You need to look at all of the information so you can make better choices that benefit you.

We have a propensity to give the medical profession a pass. We assume that they are doing everything right and that it has been tested and proved. Both being a bit of a doubting Thomas and having had a front row seat to many heart patients, I'm not impressed. So, it's a good exercise to put the practitioners of conventional medicine under the microscope and see if they are doing the right thing.

How did we get here?

Every year close to two million heart procedures are performed including bypass operations and angioplasties.

Millions of drugs are prescribed daily to the tune of billions of dollars. Still, over a half a million Americans die each year from heart disease; forty percent of those die from their *first* heart attack. Heart disease is the number one killer ahead of cancer.

It makes one wonder if all of the treatment—not to mention the "detection" and "prevention" of heart disease—is working. I don't think it is. The problem is getting worse, not better.

In the 1970s, with heart disease soaring, men in white rode in on their trusty steeds to come to the rescue. Bypass surgery became the treatment of choice and cholesterol-lowering drugs (statins) became the drugs of choice. By the late 1980s, doctors were performing over 250,000 bypass surgeries per year at a cost of over six billion dollars.[2] Today, there are over half a million done annually.[3] The medical community and the drug companies found the biggest cash cow of all time and they began to milk that baby for all it was worth.

But bypass surgery and statins were just the beginning. Angioplasty, an alternative to bypass surgery, rose to one million procedures annually in a few short years. In addition, there are now over 100 different drugs used to treat heart disease, to reduce the risk of a heart attack, or to prevent a second one if you already had one.

Was all this effective? Did it lower the incidence of heart attack and improve survival? It seems not. In 1977, a study (called "The Veterans Study") found that a group of roughly 600 patients—half of whom had bypass operations and half of whom had non-surgical care—had the same incidence of death three years later.[4] There was no difference between the bypass group and the non-bypass group. Bypass surgery provided no benefit. Unfortunately, there was such wide acceptance of these procedures that no one paid attention to this study. An even newer study in 2011 showed that drug therapy alone as good as surgery.[5] They didn't study natural therapies. I wonder why and I think you know the answer.

Later research (in the last 20 years) showed that the less invasive treatment of prescribing a beta blocker (which slows the heart down to lower blood pressure) and sending the patient home has the same results as bypass or angioplasty.[6] Even this now seems to have a long-term negative effect resulting in higher death rates. Is it really a good thing to permanently lower a patient's blood pressure to give the heart muscle less exercise?

At first, using beta blockers sounded like a plausible solution, but new research shows a different pattern emerging. In 2008, a study reported in *The American Journal of Cardiology* concluded that beta blockers "shorten your life expectancy" and cause "more heart attacks, more heart failure, and more strokes."[7] That's a frightening and sobering fact considering that millions of people are on them. Almost every single drug used to treat heart disease presents a problem ranging from increased heart risk to nutrient depletion to severe side effects sometimes resulting in death.

Standard medical treatment for symptoms

Certainly many people have benefited from and would have died without medical treatment. But studies show that conservative treatment would have, in many cases, achieved the same results. A Rand Corporation study in 1988 found up to 44 percent of bypass operations might be unneeded.[8]

How do doctors assess heart attack risk? How do they prevent heart attack? Let's look at a few different scenarios.

Scenario 1: The average person

For the average person, a routine physical gets the ball rolling. The doctor questions you about personal risk factors such as smoking, overweight, high fat diet and a sedentary lifestyle (lack of exercise). If your doctor finds high blood pressure and elevated cholesterol levels, you are told to change your diet and get more exercise. When diet and exercise fail, you are prescribed blood pressure and cholesterol lowering medication. Many people then suffer side effects—headaches, muscle pain, fatigue—and feel worse than they did *before* they started these medications. These side effects are then treated with even more drugs, which lead to more symptoms...and around and around we go.

Scenario 2: heart attack

In the worst-case scenario you suffer a heart attack. If you don't die, you receive initial treatment immediately after the heart attack to keep you alive. After stabilization in the ICU (intensive care unit) or CCU (coronary care unit), doctors usually perform bypass surgery. You then follow up with your cardiologist, who monitors the multiple medications given as aftercare.

Drugs and more drugs

Most people who have suffered a heart attack are put on four to six drugs (and some even more). The many different classes and types of drugs doctors can choose from include ACE inhibitors, beta blockers, alpha2 agonists, calcium channel blockers, diuretics, statins, anti-arrhythmics, blood thinners, and vasodilators. All of these drugs are designed to treat symptoms only.

Between generic and brand names, there are over 100 cardiac drugs out there today. Every one of these drugs, when first approved by the FDA, enjoys a 20-year patent and is sold at top dollar under its brand name. When the patent runs out, anyone can manufacture a generic form of the drug at a fraction of the price. Therefore drug companies must continually pump out new drugs to keep profits high— even if the new drugs are less effective than older drugs. These new drugs are rushed to market and often carry severe side effects. For that reason, many have been removed from the market.

This is exactly what happened in the Baycol (a calcium channel blocker) scandal. This drug caused so many deaths it was taken off the market. Even though this class of drugs is not much better than other drugs and is clearly dangerous, it is still widely prescribed today. Here's an eye opener from a December, 2000 *WebMD* news article:

> Compared with people who took other drugs, people who took calcium channel blockers to lower blood pressure had a 26% higher risk of heart attack, a 25% higher risk of heart failure, and a 10% higher risk of combined major heart disease. "Doctors should limit the use of calcium channel blockers unless other agents are not effective in lowering blood pressure or contraindicated for the patient because of side effects," says Marco Pahor M.D., professor of medicine and director of the Sticht Center on Aging at Wake Forest University School of Medicine in Winston-Salem, N.C.[9]

Another study in the December 2000 issue of *Lancet* found that compared with ACE inhibitors, calcium channel blockers increase the risk of heart disease by 19 percent and the risk of heart failure by 18 percent. That study included over 26,000 people with high blood pressure.[10] I don't know about you, but when a professor of medicine at a major university makes a statement like that in a major medical journal, I take it seriously.

Profit trumps safety

It seems that it doesn't matter that studies exposing the dangers of prescription drugs are published in prestigious scientific journals. The media machine will trot out other doctors who say the benefits outweigh the risks or cite other favorable studies. Could it possibly be that drug company profits are the motivating factor and not the benefit to the patient?

Consider this. A newer calcium channel blocker costs about $90.00 a month; an ACE inhibitor costs about $60.00 a month. Compare these with an off-patent generic diuretic at $8.00 a month. That's almost a 1000 percent difference in cost. Usually, the older and cheaper diuretic has a better track record, fewer side effects, and better results. But considering that one in four Americans suffers from high blood pressure, the drug companies stand to make billions off newer and often more dangerous drugs.

One size doesn't fit all

Something else to consider is that drugs affect ethnic groups and genders differently. Studies show that calcium channel blockers are especially dangerous for African Americans. And, it has not been determined whether they ever helped women because no women were included in the test groups. Many studies also do not include elderly patients.

The test subjects in drug studies are usually young white males. So, the recommended dosage ends up being too high for many elderly patients and they are often overdosed with the first prescription. In fact, over 120,000 deaths and over half a million serious drug reactions, which require hospitalizations, occur each year[11] from "properly" prescribed drugs, not from dosage errors.

The following graph shows that, while heart disease is the number one killer in America, prescription drugs are the fourth cause of deaths.

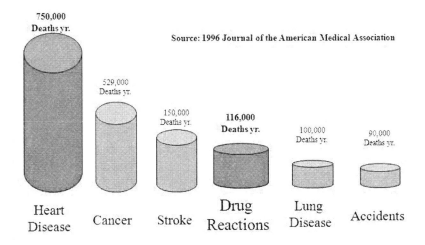

You will never see that on the nightly news...

Drugs and coenzyme Q-10

Not only do drugs increase risk of heart attack and have multiple side effects, but, as I mentioned in Chapter 1, they all cause your body to lose vitamins, minerals, and nutraceuticals. All cholesterol-lowering drugs deplete the body of coenzyme Q-10, which is essential for heart health.[12] In fact, research shows that coenzyme Q-10 is the single most important nutrient for heart muscle cells. You have to wonder why your doctor didn't tell you to take coenzyme Q-10 to replace the loss from the cholesterol-lowering drug.

I talk more about coenzyme Q-10 in Chapter 16.

If all else fails...

Of course, if nothing else lowers your blood pressure then give these medications a try. But try everything else first, such as older off patent drugs with proven track records of effectiveness and fewer side effects.

I think it's good to start with a mild diuretic and go from there. Some doctors do start with a lower dose of a diuretic for elderly patients, but this is not the norm.

Even diuretics have drawbacks; they have been shown to raise cholesterol and triglyceride levels and have side effects of weakness, muscle cramps, joint pain, and reduced libido. Diuretics also cause multiple nutrient losses including magnesium, calcium, zinc, and a host of B vitamins.

Doctors as carpenters

Allopathic (conventional medicine) doctors are in the **symptom-treating** business. Holistic doctors, like me, are in the **disease prevention** business.

There's an old saying: "If you give a carpenter a hammer, everything looks like a nail." Likewise, if you go to a surgeon you get surgery. If you go to a cardiologist you get an angioplasty. With general practitioners, you get a drug. If you go to a holistic doctor, you get nutrition and lifestyle changes.

The simple fact is, medical doctors do not have the training to recommend nutrition. And, quite frankly, they have been brainwashed by the pharmaceutical companies "drugs only" mantra. All the way from internship to clinical practice, doctors practicing conventional medicine are influenced by massive drug company advertising.

Doctors as mechanics and plumbers

Strange as it seems, the medical establishment really does look at the heart patient like a car with an engine problem. In this mechanical model, your heart is the pump, the blood vessels are hoses, and the kidneys are the filters. Drugs are used to slow down the heart to reduce stress, open the hoses (blood vessels), and increase fluid loss from the kidneys to reduce pressure. Angioplasty is designed to open any artery blockages. Bypass surgery reroutes the blood around the blockage.

If you have a blockage in the coronary arteries (blood vessels to the heart) they put in new vessels. It's a plumbing problem. If the arteries are blocked, put in some new pipes (vessels) that go around the blockage.

Hopping on the drug treadmill

As I mentioned previously, if you are diagnosed with heart disease or end up in the hospital—in which instance you probably had a bypass—you will end up taking on average four to six drugs as your aftercare program.

If you visit your doctor for a routine checkup and have high blood pressure or elevated cholesterol levels, you might get the same number of medications.

If your doctor does a routine EKG that shows any abnormalities, he can start you on some medications but usually refers you to a cardiologist or the nearest emergency room. The cardiologist can do an angiogram right in his office. If the angiogram shows any blockage, you get either a balloon angioplasty or he refers you to the hospital where a cardiac surgeon does a bypass operation. Either way, the aftercare is still the handful of medications you must take for life.

Standard procedure is to give a cholesterol-lowering drug (statin) and two or three blood pressure drugs. Usually beta blockers are given to slow the heart down, causing it to pump slower and with less stress. A diuretic is added to further lower blood pressure by flushing water from the kidneys. Again, these drugs are just treating the symptoms. There are no good research studies to prove that treating "risk factors" will actually stop or prevent heart attacks. Cholesterol lowering medications help only if you already have advanced heart disease.

Caution: If you experience new symptoms, always attribute them to the new drug until proven otherwise. Many times a new drug will be prescribed for the new symptoms when, in fact, the symptoms are a result of the drugs you are already taking.

So what are doctors doing to reverse heart disease? Sorry to say, nothing. In many cases, if the medical establishment only stops you from getting worse, they consider this a victory.

Do people really do better with the plumbing job approach? A noted epidemiologist, Dr. Charles T. McGee M.D., does not think so. In his book *Heart Fraud: Uncovering the Biggest Health Scam in History* (Piccadilly Books, 2007), Dr. McGee attacks the entire gamut of cardiac procedures, from bypass surgery to drug therapy.

Artery blockage: two options

If you experience chest pains—a sign of not enough blood getting to the heart—immediate medical attention is needed. Most people are referred to a cardiologist or to the ER. The cardiologist performs a series of tests starting with a stress test, which involves running on a treadmill while hooked up to an EKG machine.

If the results are abnormal the cardiologist performs an angiogram. He or she makes an incision into your thigh and threads a catheter up the femoral artery into your heart. A dye is then injected and pictures are taken to see if there are any artery blockages. If there is blockage, the cardiologist has two options:

- Perform angioplasty.
- Perform bypass surgery.

Door #1: angioplasty

With angioplasties, there are two methods:

- A balloon angioplasty.
- A balloon angioplasty with a stent.

In a balloon angioplasty, the cardiologist threads a balloon into the artery to the point of blockage and inflates it, opening up the artery.

Many times the artery closes back down, so the doctor places a metal mesh, called a stent, inside the artery to keep it open. But even with metal stents in place, the coronary arteries still often close up. Newer drug-emitting stents (stents coated with drugs) have been used in an effort to stop the arteries from closing. Despite research results, which show that the

Caution: If you have any symptoms such as shortness of breath or chest or arm pain, dial 911 or go the nearest emergency room. Never delay or self treat. You can always seek alternative care via natural methods later to deal with your aftercare and long-term management.

new stents are not as good as had been predicted, they are used nonetheless.

Although there is risk with angioplasty (some people die from a reaction to the dye that is injected to make the artery blockage visible), there are more risks with the coronary artery bypass surgery. Many patients are sold on angioplasty because they have a natural fear of going to the hospital and having a major operation. These procedures are less invasive and can be done right in the doctor's office. You go home the same day. They are cheaper than—and some say as effective as—a bypass operation. Recovery is also much quicker, so you don't have to spend a few weeks in the hospital.

The problem with angioplasty is that, many times, the artery closes up within months of the procedure requiring the procedure to be repeated, which increases risk of a severe reaction or death. Former Vice-President Dick Cheney is a classic example of this.

Door #2: bypass surgery

The second option is to have a bypass surgery, formally called a coronary artery bypass graft (or CABG, referred to as "cabbage"). With this surgery, they open you up and graft veins from other parts of your body. The harvested veins are used to reroute blood flow around the blockage. Grafts last five to ten years and then you need to have them redone.

They usually harvest the veins from your legs. Newer techniques, however, use veins from your chest, which seems to work just as well or better. And an advantage to using chest veins is that you don't have enormous scars on your legs afterwards.

Afterwards, the doctor usually tells that you were lucky he caught it and that you were a walking dead man or woman. They refer to these blockages as "widow makers." It seems as if it's always a "90 percent blockage and you could drop dead if the bypass isn't done right away." It scares you to out of your mind and into surgery.

This is exactly what happened to Sharon, 58. "I went to the doctor and the next thing I knew I was admitted to the hospital and had a bypass operation. I think it was unneeded, and now I'm on a slew of drugs that make me feel lethargic and not myself anymore."

Again, back to the plumber analogy. The sewage is backed up because a pipe is blocked. The plumber/doctor bypasses the blockage with another pipe to get the sewage/blood flowing again.

With bypass surgery, there is a chance of death due to serious complications in 1 to 4% percent of cases. It is very expensive and recovery is painful and takes several weeks.

Door #1? Or Door #2?

Comparing bypass to angioplasty, a March 2009 study found that bypass worked better in the short run, but had the same results—except for an unwanted increase in the number of strokes—in the long term (after twelve months) as angioplasty.[13]

There is good evidence, though, that people who have had heart attacks do better with bypass when three blood vessels are blocked. Still, if you are being treated for chest pains, drugs work just as well without the complications and risks associated with surgery or angioplasty.

Fuzzy math and drug companies

Fuzzy math creates deception. When you talk about drugs and how effective they are, you have to understand the secret language of the drug companies and scientists who do the studies. You must know the mathematical terms or you will think you're taking a wonderful drug that will save your life when, in fact, nothing could be further from the truth. The terms you need to know are:

- Number needed to treat (NNT).
- Absolute risk (AR).
- Relative risk number (RR).
- Number needed to harm (NNTH).

NNT (number needed to treat)

NNT represents the number of people who have to take a drug to prevent one outcome. Many times, 50 to 200 people must take a drug for three to five years to prevent only a very few actual events.

So, if I told you that a drug helped only one in 100 who took it, you wouldn't be very impressed. But many drugs do, indeed, help only one in 100.

Take the case of aspirin: Over 300 women must take aspirin for four years to prevent one stroke. The one less stroke for every 314 women who take aspirin for four years is a terrible tradeoff as many more will have bleeding ulcers and some will have brain hemorrhages due to the blood being too thin and not clotting. This 314 to 1 ratio is the number needed to treat (NNT).

The NNT for cholesterol lowering drugs is 100. One hundred people must take a statin for three years to prevent one non-fatal heart attack at a cost of around $260,000.

AR (absolute risk)

The AR is the number of events (good or bad) in a treated or control group divided by the number of people in that group. For example, 100 people took a drug and there were two heart attacks. One hundred people took a placebo (sugar pill) and there were three heart attacks. The difference is one person or one percent.

RRN (relative risk number)

Now, here comes the fuzzy math part. Instead of using the NNT or the AR, drug companies devised a number called relative risk (RR). RR is the measure of the relative success of one treatment as opposed to another. So in our example, the difference between two and three hearts attacks is 33 percent (a fraction of the number of people who had a heart attack divided by the number who didn't).

So, a one percent reduction in heart attacks turns into an advertisement claiming a 33 percent reduction. That sounds better. Clever, don't you think? Criminal comes to mind.

By the way, a study showed that when doctors were informed of the AR of a drug compared to the RR, they wouldn't prescribe the drug to their patients.

NNTH (number needed to harm)

The number needed to harm (NNTH) is important, too, as it represents the number of people who must take the drug for harm to occur or to cause an adverse outcome. These numbers are usually high, such as 1000 or 2500, but that means that for every 1000 or more people who take the drug, one is detrimental and may result in death.

Sometimes a drug will show lower incidence of a condition but also shows a higher death rate for those who took the drug. You need to know the total death rate from taking the drug, not just the lowering of the condition.

So the lesson here is, before you take a drug, ask your doctor what the NNT, the AR, and the NNTH of the drug is, not the RR. And let's not forget the total mortality and morbidity (actual increase in death rates from using a drug).

The deception of "proven" surgery

Another disturbing factor that many consumers are unaware of is that surgical techniques are not thoroughly tested before they go into widespread practice. Many procedures gain wide acceptance without ever being tested. This is what happened with stents.[14] Stents were used on the conjecture that the procedure was superior to bypass or drug therapy alone, but no testing was done to confirm that hypothesis. The FDA approved stents on the basis that a follow up study would be done as the original research was done off shore (in another country). Of course no follow up study was done to date.

And although stents were not thoroughly tested they were, nevertheless, aggressively marketed to physicians. The entire stent industry relied on a few studies that were never repeated for accuracy as required by the FDA. Why? It's a big money maker for drug companies who make stents and for cardiologists who can do the procedure right in the office. The cardiologist, who didn't do bypass surgery before and would have to refer the patient to a cardiac surgeon, now could insert the stent through the same catheter already in place from the angiogram and make a good profit.

Is it really a surprise, then, that stent use climbed to over one million a year in only ten years? Stents, by the way, were supposed to be tested in more double blind controlled studies but never were.

Expensive antibiotics, anyone?

Here's another great idea that was never tested but went into standard practice making the drug companies a bundle. When pathologists studied plaque removed from arteries they found there was bacterium present called *chlamydia pneumonia.* They theorized that this bacterium was responsible for the rupturing of the atherosclerotic plaque leading to the heart attack. As a result, every heart patient was given very expensive bag of antibiotics while in intensive care.

This went on for years until a study was finally done to see if the theory was correct. Researchers found the bacterium to be an innocent bystander and the antibiotics did nothing to prevent or treat the heart attack. They looked at 11 studies involving over 19,217 patients and concluded:

> "Evidence available to date does not demonstrate **an overall benefit of antibiotic therapy in reducing mortality or cardiovascular events in patients with CAD** [Coronary Artery Disease]."[15]

Oops. We *thought* it was a good idea. Antibiotics are no longer standard procedure.

The risk factor game

If you know the 1970 movie, *Catch-22*, you not only show your age, but you remember this parody of the tragedy of war. In the movie, pilots desperately wanted out of a war and asked to be relieved from duty because they were insane. The catch? If they were insane they couldn't fly. But since they were flying they were obviously sane. Therefore they could never get out of flying because they weren't insane.

The heart disease "risk factor game" uses the same circular logic. You are told that you must lower your risk factors of having a heart attack. But will that prevent a heart attack? No, but you have to lower your risk factors associated with a heart attack...

Smoke screen

Of the major risk factors—the only one with any great reliability in reducing heart disease and stroke—is smoking. We all know that. If you smoke, stop. It's probably one of the best things you can do for your health. The other major risk factors are high blood pressure, high cholesterol, being overweight, and lack of exercise.

At this point, you might be asking, "Dr. Pilgreen, do you mean to tell me that the risk factors I continually hear about are not that important? It's just smoke and mirrors?" No. By reducing risk factors some people—not all—do have fewer heart attacks. Many people with risk factors do not have heart attacks. For example, Winston Churchill, who was famously overweight and smoked, lived to the ripe old age of 90. On the other hand, James Fixx, a famous runner who wrote books on health and running, died of a massive coronary at the age of 52.

It's a catch-22. By lowering the risk factors you should be lowering risk, but that's not always the case.

Aspirin and other blood thinners

Aspirin: the be all and end all of drugs. We've all seen the TV ads that claim that aspirin prevents heart attacks and that everyone should take them. One a day whether you need it or not.

But these wonder drug pushers were dealt a blow by a drug advisory panel when it found aspirin was not all it was cracked up to be. The panel looked at the effectiveness of daily aspirin intake in reducing heart attacks and found that it would reduce only eight heart attacks for every 1000 people who took it daily over five years. The same number of people would have three hemorrhagic strokes and one death due to gastrointestinal bleeding. That means that 1 person in 125 (NNT) would not have a non-fatal heart attack, but 1 in 250 (NNTH) would have a stroke or die from an ulcer. That doesn't seem like a good trade off.

Aspirin and women

According to a large study published in the *New England Journal of Medicine*, there is no benefit in aspirin consumption for prevention of heart attacks or death from heart attacks in women. The study showed only a lowered risk of stroke. How many women do you know who take an aspirin a day to prevent a heart attack?

This really is a "choose your poison" issue. Aspirin will reduce the types of stroke you get from a blood clot but it will increase the number of strokes from brain bleeding. Aspirin causes many hospitalizations from bleeding stomach ulcers and even death.

Aspirin and men

Aspirin does help in men who have had heart attacks and have serious heart disease, but not in men with normal risk factors. In fact, it has proven ineffective in reducing heart attacks or death: 155 (NNT) men had to take the aspirin for five years to prevent one non-fatal heart attack. There were, however, more bleeding type strokes and stomach hemorrhages. Aspirin is nothing to trifle with. It can cause bleeding leading to stroke or ulcers requiring hospitalization. Let me tell you the story John a golfer who ended up having to wear diapers because he was bleeding from the rectum was so severe. Rectal bleeding is not good as you think of polyps, hemorrhoids or even cancer. After extensive testing, doctors found that an 81 mg baby aspirin was the culprit. I have another patient who had the same problem. Aspirin consumption is not without risks. Carefully consider the options before taking aspirin everyday with your doctor.

Plavix to the rescue

Plavix (generic name clopidogrel) is purported to prevent blood clots and is often prescribed for people who face an increased risk for heart attacks and strokes. Take a look at this chart:

Clopidogrel Sulfate Tablets (Plavix)

The curves showing the overall event rate are shown in Figure 1. The event curves separated early and continue to diverge over the three year follow up period.

Fatal or Non-Fatal Vascular Events in the CAPRIE Study

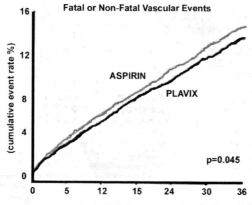

Although the statistical signifigance favoring Plavix over Aspirin was marginal (P=0.045), and represents the result of a single trial that has not been replicated, the comparator drug Aspirin is itself effective (vs. palcebo) in reducing cardiovascular events in patients with recent myocardial infarctrion or stroke. Thus, the difference between Plavix and placebo although not measured directly, is substantial.

(Note: The above text is omitted from the official website.)

The chart shows that there is absolutely no difference in effects of aspirin compared to Plavix. The greatest difference is that a tablet of aspirin cost a half of a cent, while Plavix is $6.00 a pill.

There are currently a lot of commercials about Plavix, and it's prescribed like water. Plavix is the number two drug prescribed with over $9 billion in sales as of 2008. However, there are a few problems...

Plavix irritates the stomach lining so it has to be taken in conjunction with proton pump inhibitors (PPIs). These include omeprazole (Prilosec and Zegerid), lansoprazole (Prevacid), pantoprazole (Protonix), rabeprazole (Aciphex) and esomeprazole (Nexium). But when you mix the two you increase the number of heart attacks.

Plavix does not work on certain patients and leads to more heart attacks, especially in people who have had stents implanted. A study showed that 40 percent of European Americans, 40 percent of African ancestry and 50 percent of Asian ancestry don't fare well. That's 80 percent of the American population.

A study published by the *New England Journal of Medicine* showed that, for people who were at high risk of heart attack and for those who had already had a heart attack, taking Plavix showed no benefit. When they looked at low risk patients who took the drug, there was an **increase** in heart attack, stroke and death—not exactly what they had hoped for.[16] The study also said that Plavix "caused higher death rates when taking both aspirin and Plavix."[17]

Finally, the FDA just recently found Plavix to be so dangerous and ineffective that it will require a black box warning—the severest FDA warning allowed. In spite of these results, Plavix is still the number one drug prescribed worldwide. And the commercials never seem to cease.

Wizard of Oz

When you challenge the medical/drug establishment with their own research results by pointing to non-existent or harmful results of drug treatment, you get a variety of responses. They claim that longer term use will show benefits or that more data is needed. Here's a standard list they trot out every time they are called out:

- The drugs have fewer side effects than other drugs.
- The drugs have better results than other drugs even with side effects.
- We did put a warning on it (a black box warning).
- Studies were done on the wrong kind of patients; others could benefit but we need more studies.
- The study shows negative results because of the author's publication bias.

On the other hand, vitamins nearly always get a bad rap. You will hardly ever find any sustained positive reporting of a good result from vitamins, but you will always have negative results plastered all over the media.

Commonly prescribed heart medications

Let's look at some studies that highlight the dangers of many commonly prescribed classes of heart medications taken by millions of Americans.

Beta blockers

Beta blockers are a class of heart drugs that slow the heart muscle down by inhibiting the electrical impulses to the beta-adergenic portion of the nerves. There are over 22 different beta blockers on the market, but one of the most widely prescribed is Atenolol. In the November 6, 2004 issue of *Lancet*, Dr. Bo Carlberg and colleagues at Umea University Hospital in Sweden reviewed several studies and found that Atenolol is not as effective as a placebo (sugar pill) and, in fact, it increases heart disease deaths, incidence of stroke, and overall death rates.[18] So, why is it one of the most frequently prescribed drugs on the market for heart disease? Beats me.

ACE inhibitors

ACE inhibitors are a class of drugs that block an enzyme produced by the kidney that raises blood pressure by constricting blood vessels. The kidneys need pressure to filter the blood and secrete angiotension II to constrict the blood vessels and raise blood pressure. ACE inhibitors block this enzyme.

ACE inhibitors and many other drugs are needed in the acute phase, but long-term use causes problems unless the underlying cause is addressed. Even though the number needed to treat is 50 or more, it is recommended to all patients as the following EUROPA Study published in the medical journal *Lancet* concluded:

> Among patients with stable coronary heart disease without apparent heart failure, perindopril [ACE inhibitor] can significantly improve outcome. About 50 patients need to be treated for a period of 4 years to prevent one major cardiovascular event. Treatment with perindopril, on top of other preventive medications, should be considered in all patients with coronary heart disease.[19]

So, in people with pre-existing heart disease but without heart failure, the drug will prevent a heart attack in only one out of 50 people who took it for four years. Therefore, it is recommended that it be given to everybody with coronary artery disease. If an antibiotic worked on one in 50 people we would think that was insane. This drug doesn't work very well, does it?

If a vitamin had the same results, the medical establishment would not recommend it. It would be considered too expensive and of little benefit. But if a drug works this poorly, they give it to millions of patients to the tune of billions of dollars and tout it as the best thing since sliced bread.

Calcium channel blockers

Calcium channel blockers are newer heart drugs that work by blocking calcium to the heart muscle cells to slow the rate of contraction. Again, this is the mechanical model of slowing the heart down to take stress off the heart muscle.

Because older off-patent drugs such as beta blockers, ACE inhibitors, and diuretics can be made as generics and sold at greatly reduced prices, newer more expensive drugs are created even if they cause more harm than good. This is exactly the case with calcium channel blockers. They have a terrible track record and have serious side effects and can cause death. Here is what Dr. Marco Pahor, Professor of Medicine and Director of the Sticht Center on Aging at Wake Forest University School of Medicine in Winston-Salem, NC, and colleagues had to say about calcium-channel blockers after studying close to 30,000 people from over nine different studies who took them:[20]

> In randomized controlled trials, the large available database suggests that calcium antagonists are inferior to other types of antihypertensive drugs as first-line agents in reducing the risks of several major complications of hypertension. On the basis of these data, the longer-acting calcium antagonists cannot be recommended as first-line therapy for hypertension.

In addition, the article stressed that they are perfectly good and useful drugs and shouldn't be considered harmful. How can they say that this drug can kill you or cause serious harm from an adverse reaction and then turn right around in the same paper and still say the drug is useful? That directly contradicts the facts of the research. The study shows that those taking this class of drugs had an increase in heart attacks and congestive heart failure. Not exactly the side affects you are looking for when treating high blood pressure, one of the primary reasons they are prescribed. To be fair, there are some experts that think calcium channel blockers are the best drugs to use for high blood pressure over diuretics, which have their own problems. I say, natural first and then drugs as a last resort. Or, drugs, and then transition to natural care.

Bestsellers

There are over a hundred drugs that are prescribed for heart disease. Here are the top sellers:

- Lipitor (cholesterol lowering) is number one with over $10 billion in sales and 70 million prescriptions.
- Lisinopril (ACE inhibitor, lowers blood pressure) with 45 million prescriptions.
- Atenolol (beta blocker for blood pressure) with 44 million prescriptions.
- Hydrochlorothiazide (diuretic) with 41 million prescriptions.
- Zocor (cholesterol) with $6 billion in sales and 30 million prescriptions.
- Norvasc (amlodipine, calcium channel blocker) with $4.5 billion in sales and 35 million prescriptions.
- Plavix (blood thinner) with $9 billion in sales worldwide as of 2008 and 20 million prescriptions in the United States.

The polypill pushers

In 2003, Professor Nicholas Wald, head of London's Wolfson Institute of Preventive Medicine and his colleague, Professor Malcolm Law of the University of Auckland in New Zealand, published their case for the prevention of heart disease using a "polypill." A polypill contains multiple medications with the goal of reducing the number of pills that need to be taken.

Their pill had a statin, three blood pressure drugs (beta blocker, ACE inhibitor, and diuretic), 0.8 milligrams of folic acid, and aspirin. This is insane considering all the side effects, nutrient loss, and the lack of success of these drugs.

In another study, these same professors concluded that everyone—whether you have high blood pressure or not—should take blood pressure lowering drugs. Dr. Franz Messerli of St. Luke's-Roosevelt Hospital Center, New York City, had this response to the study design and conclusions:

> They combined 147 trials in their meta-analysis to make numerous assumptions, some possibly valid, others clearly not. Numerous meta-analyses have clearly demonstrated that beta blockers do not reduce the risk of coronary heart disease in hypertension, despite the fact that they lower blood pressure. Thus, despite its appearance of being bigger and better, this study is yet another example of my dictum: "A meta-analysis is like a sausage, only God and the butcher know what goes in it and neither would ever eat any."

Well said.

But everybody's doing it...

Again, my goal isn't to pummel the drug establishment, but there is so much darn dirty laundry. There has been almost a total loss of trust in medical research and reporting. It started about six years ago with one doctor getting caught giving a positive review for a new drug and publishing it in the *Journal of the American Medical Association*. It was later found that the doctor had received money from the drug company, a clear conflict of interest.

This shocked the medical community and there was going to be hell to pay...or was there? A subsequent study showed that when doctors receive money or perks from a drug company and review a drug, the reviews are positive 70 percent of the time. When they are not compensated, the reviews are positive only 40 percent of the time.

In fact, so many doctors had been compromised that the major medical journals were suspect. They lost a lot of credibility. But they recovered. How? They cried foul and claimed, "Everybody was doing it." In fact, it seems that all phases of research and development were compromised.

Research done at the National Institutes of Health (the big government bureaucracy that we taxpayers fund) was totally infested with such deals. Some of the goodies? Free luxury trips, paid speaking engagements, cash (honoraria), high paying consulting fees and—my personal favorite— stock options. It seems that everybody was on the take.

Congressional hearings were held and panels created to sort out the problem.

The solution? Drum roll please...

The solution: Government funded researchers, private journals, and researchers at major universities need to have the help and oversight of drug companies. Really? Isn't this the fox guarding the hen house?

Here's their rationale. Researchers claimed that they can't do the research unless the drug companies pay for it. And, because drug companies fund the research, they have control over when and how the data is collected and disseminated. Of course, they deny this and say that they have non-biased panels that review the data. But, ultimately, they have control over the final draft.

They also determined that it's okay to accept drug company funding and oversight, but the doctors doing the studies must include a disclaimer stating who funded the study or what monetary compensation had been received— whether working on the study or writing a review. You see these disclaimers today in almost all studies published in major medical journals.

The coup de grace is ghostwriting. That is, someone else writes the study and the scientist or doctor supposedly checks what is written and signs off on it. The ghostwriter is paid by those with a vested interest in casting the drug in the best light. Many times, the person writing or editing the study omits negative information while pumping up the positives, even to the point of lying.

A case in point is Vioxx. This "revolutionary" pain killer didn't have the side effect of bleeding ulcers that had plagued long term users of aspirin and ibuprofen. Vioxx was a pain killer touted as the next best thing since the invention of the automobile. One thing the ghostwriter failed to mention in the study, however, was that Vioxx increased heart attacks. Yikes. Most doctors won't prescribe Vioxx now unless nothing else is working.

Paroxatine (Paxil) is another example. Paroxatine is prescribed to treat depression, obsessive-compulsive disorder, and anxiety. In a review, a ghostwriter said that the drug was effective and useful for pediatric care. The research results, however, showed it was not effective and caused harm. Doctors names on the study gave it credibility.

Now we are left to wonder whether the research can be trusted at all. In three of the last four studies I have cited, over 30 percent of the participants dropped out. Other studies showed that over 40 percent did not take the drug. Most research is still done only on young white males. So not only is the research biased, but it is many times falsified.

The bottom line

The *Journal of the American Medical Association* published a study in 1998 documenting the large number of people dying from adverse drug reactions. The study showed that prescription drugs were the fourth leading cause of death in the United States right behind heart disease and cancer.[21] The study also exposed the fact that 2.2 million people had serious drug reactions while in the hospital. An earlier study in 1997 demonstrated that if you went to the hospital and had an adverse drug reaction (ADR), you had double the chance of dying.[22]

What this means to you and me is that we should never take a drug until it's been on the market for over two years. For the last eight years I have cautioned people to wait when a new drug comes on the market.

If you must take drugs, the best advice is to always use older off patent drugs that have a good track record. Start with the lowest dose possible and with the least number of drugs. You can always increase the dosage or add drugs but you can't reverse a serious side effect. There are hundreds of thousands of serious adverse side effects that can result from taking a medication properly prescribed by a doctor just once—and in some cases the side affect is death. Be very cautious and get your doctor to try more non-invasive procedures and fewer drugs if at all possible.

A happy side note: A blue ribbon panel was recently commissioned by the government to study the problems with the FDA approval process since so many dangerous drugs were getting to market. The panel exceeded my wait-and-see position and recommended that the dreaded black box warning be on all new drugs for the first two years to catch any serious problems.

Beyond the drugs: do your own research

Don't be afraid to challenge your doctor. Ask tough questions such as: "How long am I going to be on this drug?" and "Are there effective drugs with fewer side effects?"

Show your doctor this book. Point to the studies. Your doctor has a computer and can look them up. So can you.

- W**ww.pub-med.org**, a government database that contains all drug research and is free to the public.
- If you're concerned about a drug, go to **www.drugs.com**.
- If you want to know about lab tests such hs-CRP or lipoprotein-a (discussed in Chapter 5), go to **www.labonline.com**.

It's your life and your body. Be proactive. Educate yourself. This book is a great start. Always try to sift through the rhetoric on both sides. I don't want to end up as another statistic and I'm guessing you don't either.

Enough with the bad and scary news. Let's get to what you can do to inform and protect yourself.

3

The Truth about Cholesterol

"Endarteritis Deformans Atheroma (plaque)
is a product of an inflammatory process
within the intima (artery wall)."

— Rudolph Virchow (1821-1902)
The Father of Modern Pathology

N othing is more controversial than the cholesterol theory of heart disease. I call it the FEAR (false evidence appearing real) theory. The cholesterol theory has been around for over 60 years—ever since a doctor showed that feeding rabbits mountains of trans fats caused plaque to build up on the animals' arteries. That was followed by the Framingham heart study that showed people with higher cholesterol levels suffered more heart attacks.

The drug companies' solution was to lower cholesterol levels by blocking production in the body. Problem solved, right? Not so fast. Over 20 studies were done over the next 30 years to prove this theory, but only one showed a positive effect. No matter, cholesterol lowering medications are now a 65 billion dollar a year business and, by golly, scientific facts are not going to get in the way of profit.

The real cause: inflammation

The truth is that inflammation is the cause of artery disease, not cholesterol. The only reason that cholesterol lowering drugs work at all is that they lower inflammation, not by lowering cholesterol levels. And cholesterol lowering drugs are only beneficial to those who have already had heart attacks, but not to those without preexisting heart disease.

I mentioned a study in Chapter 2 that claims that statins are good for everybody to take, even those without heart disease. Believe it or not, some want to put statins into the water supply. This makes me crazy. There are many side effects, increases in diabetes, and overall death rates caused by statins.

The newest study, JUPITOR, is touted as the conclusive evidence that statins work. The group in that study, by the way, was stacked with people who have inflammation, were overweight, and prone to heart disease—just the type of people who are not supposed to be in the study of that nature. When the final tally came in, there was not a 46 percent relative risk reduction in heart attacks, but a paltry one percent absolute risk reduction. Additionally, there was a doubling of diabetes in the treated group which the researchers said was insignificant. Diabetes is not an insignificant complication.

In the case of the statin Lipitor, over 100 men must take it for three years to prevent one non-fatal heart attack at a cost of $260,000.00. That is a 99 percent failure rate and a whale of a price tag.

Blocking cholesterol production in the body is an absurd idea when you understand that cholesterol is needed by almost every cell in the body. If you don't eat cholesterol, your body will produce it.

The following chart shows that every hormone—male, female, and adrenal—is synthesized from cholesterol.

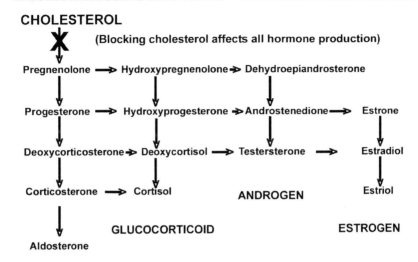

Cholesterol as dogma

It's a scientific fact that inflammation causes heart disease. That fact is not disputed by those who have read the current research. It's frustrating to me, however, because the idea that excess cholesterol causes heart disease has risen to the level of religious dogma (on the part of drug companies and the media). Billions of dollars of advertising has brainwashed both the public and the medical profession.

Unfortunately, the drug companies have put all their eggs in one basket and continue trying to make the research fit. I say, if the research doesn't fit then you need to quit. The bad news for us all is that they will not quit until everyone is drinking the Kool-Aid (also known as, the drugs).

Now, there is one benefit in cholesterol lowering drugs. They do lower inflammation by stopping some of the inflammatory substances produced by the body, but not all. They do not work by lowering cholesterol levels.

The fact is, there has been a threefold increase in congestive heart failure since statins have been unleashed. People over 65 with the lowest cholesterol levels have the highest death rates. You need cholesterol as you get older.

Size matters

Blocking all cholesterol does not fix the problem. The type of cholesterol in the body is more important than the amount.

Lipoprotein-a (LP-A) are bullet-sized particles—called remnant lipoprotein (RLP)— that pierce the vessel lining and start the plaque process. They include dangerous HDL3 (high density lipoprotein) particles. The smaller the particle size the greater the risk.

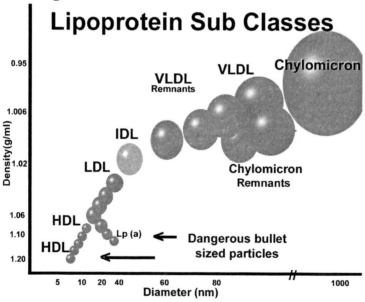

The above chart shows the many sizes and kinds of cholesterol particles—from the very large chylomicron size particles to the very small Lp(a) and HDL3. These Lp(a) particles are small, dense, and cause severe damage to the artery lining causing the plaque process.

If your cholesterol levels are normal but you have an abundance of small cholesterol particles in your body, you are in danger of a heart attack. Your cholesterol can be low but if the majority is the Lp-A particles, you are in big trouble. This is the classic case of a person going to the doctor and getting a clean bill of health only to die the next day of a massive heart attack. It's like a tennis net. The tennis ball (normal-sized particle) will not go through the net, but a golf ball (small-sized particle) will. The good news is, to lower the number of small-sized particles, take a balanced supplement, niacin, and fish oils.

Your body needs cholesterol

You need cholesterol to produce vitamin D, absorb minerals, make hormones, needed to make nerve and brain cells, and it's a component of all cell membranes. Blocking cholesterol produces side effects of memory loss, muscle pain, fatigue, rhabidomyosis (muscle breakdown that can lead to death), an increase in death rates (especially in the elderly), and liver disease. I have two patients who suffered hair loss due to statins, but were assured that the drug was not the cause. Hmmm. I beg to differ.

Further reading

You can learn more history and scientific facts about cholesterol from the following books:
- *The Cholesterol Myth*, by Uffe Ravenskov, M.D., Ph.D.
- *Hidden Truth about Cholesterol-Lowering Drugs*, by Shane Ellison, M.Sc.

- *Heart Frauds*, by Charles T. McGee, M.D.
- *Malignant Medical Myths*, by Joel M. Kaufman, Ph.D.

Keep in mind, though, that while all these books expose the cholesterol myth, they are outdated as new research shows the real cause is inflammation.

Getting to the root cause

I know that many of you will ignore my warning and continue to take the cholesterol lowering drugs because you are afraid not to. Rightfully so. But know that the only way to treat heart disease is to treat the root cause—inflammation caused by faulty diet, inadequate nutrient intake, and a toxic environment. So, even if you elect to take medication you must replace the nutrients that the drug depletes from your body as well as those that are needed to reverse heart disease.

Nutrients are the only solution. Olive oil, fish oil, niacin, and a balanced supplement are what I recommend to my patients. You need to include coenzyme Q-10 to replace the loss from statins. I talk more about coenzyme Q-10 in chapter 15.

Statins also damage muscle cells (called statin-induced muscle toxicity) causing muscle pain and fatigue in a majority of patients due to a depletion of the amino acid carnitine. Carnitine must be taken when on statins to prevent this muscle deterioration. I will talk about carntine more in chapter 6.

Taking these nutrients not only lowers cholesterol levels, but changes the size and number of particles. In fact, nutrients are the only treatment for these types of particles. The following chart shows how the process works.

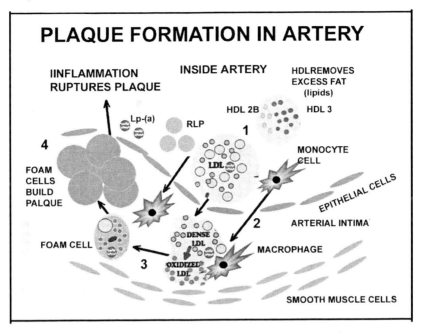

PLAQUE FORMATION IN ARTERY

1. Inflammatory substances damage the lining of the blood vessel wall allowing remnant lipoprotein Lp(a) to pierce the vessel wall.

2. The body sends in white blood cells (macrophages) to eat up the foreign bodies (cholesterol particles).

3. This gooey mess of debris turns into a foam cell.

4. The plaque builds up on the foam cell and it pushes into the vessel wall causing the blocking of the artery.

5. A fibrous cap forms on top and can break off, sending a clot to the heart and causing a heart attack by blocking a coronary artery.

So, inflammation is the cause of artery damage, followed by the infiltration of bad cholesterol, not the amount of cholesterol in the body.

There are many inflammatory substances that cause the damage to the epithelial lining of the blood vessels. Cholesterol drugs neutralize a few of them, and are the reason they work at all—not by the lowering of cholesterol levels.

Stopping all inflammatory byproducts with nutrients are more effective and have no adverse sides effects like weakness, fatigue, muscle pain, rhabibomyosis, or liver damage associated with statins.

The next chart shows cholesterol size does matter in the plaque process. Also, there are many inflammatory products that cause damage to the lining of the blood vessel wall. This chart shows just five (adhesion molecules, PAI-1, MCP-1, colony stimulating factors and tissue factor) of the over 20 substances that damage the blood vessel lining. This is the newest research by the scientific community. There's quite a bit more biochemistry and I have simplified the graph to make it easier to understand. We are all under great inflammatory assault on our blood vessels from our diet and environment.

Cholesterol (Lipoproteins) size and Atherosclerosis

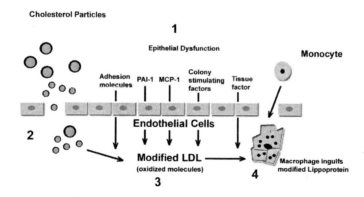

1. The epithelial lining is damaged by the inflammatory cytokines.

2. The small remnant cholesterol particles enter into the damaged vessel wall.

3. The inflammatory cytokines oxidize the cholesterol (LDL).

4. The macrophage engulfs the modified (LDL) lipoprotein.

To prevent this process, I recommend using nutrition, along with the drugs, and try to wean yourself off (with your doctor's approval, of course) of them. If your current doctor won't agree, try finding one that is more holistically minded.

Natural nutrients and nutraceuticals, along with diet and exercise are the only real lasting methods of reversing artery damage.

4

Drugs and Nutrient Loss

"Whenever a doctor cannot do good, he must be kept from doing harm."

— *Hippocrates*

Heart disease is progressive so you need a concentrated effort of diet, exercise, and supplements to combat it. And then there are drugs. Please don't misunderstand me. Drugs in some cases can have disastrous consequences, but they are useful and necessary in **initial treatment**. Thank God we have them.

Drugs, however, should be used with extreme caution and only for short periods until natural therapy has taken hold. Your goal should be to get weaned off them if at all possible.

Of course, some people must be on drugs long term. Long-term drug use, however, causes nutrient depletion and many times increases heart disease—the exact thing they are supposed to treat. For instance, Hydralazine, a vasodilator, causes more heart disease than it's trying to correct. You cannot put a toxic drug in the body that poisons an enzyme system or blocks an important metabolic pathway without having long-term negative side effects.

The following table shows the most commonly taken drugs to treat cardiovascular disease, the nutrients depleted, and side effects. No wonder many people who take these drugs felt worse after they started treatment!

Commonly Used Drugs to Treat Heart Disease

Drug/Procedure	Prescribed For	Side Effects
Statins[*]	Lowering cholesterol	Memory loss, irritability, nerve and muscle pain, congestive heart failure, depletes the body of coenzyme Q-10
Ace inhibitors[**]	Lowering blood pressure	Chronic cough in 10% who take them, kidney problems and rash. Zinc depletion
Beta blockers	Slowing heart rate; lowering blood pressure	May injure the lining of the blood vessels, increases heart attack risk, and causes nutrient coenzyme Q-10 and melatonin depletion
Calcium channel blockers	Slowing the rate of heart muscle contraction	Increases heart attacks, heart disease, and the risk of heart failure and calcium depletion.
Diuretics	Lowering blood pressure	Increases cholesterol and triglyceride levels, weakness, muscle cramps, joint pain, reduced libido, loss of nutrients: magnesium, calcium, zinc, B-vitamins

*Ineffective for women, people over 65, and people who have never had a heart attack.
**Reduces the chance of heart attack to one in 50.

Adding up the nutrient loss

As I mentioned previously, the average cardiac patient is on four or more drugs:

- Something to make the heart pump more forcefully (cardiac glycoside-Digoxin).
- Something to slow the heart down (beta blocker).
- Something to lower the blood pressure by stopping the kidneys from secreting an enzyme that normally raises it (ACE inhibitor)
- A diuretic to make the kidneys lose even more fluid to further lower blood pressure
- Oh, and almost all heart patients are put on cholesterol lowering drugs whether they need them or not.
- And aspirin, to boot.

Add this up and you'll see why people feel tired, have less energy, don't sleep well, and suffer more anxiety and depression from nutrient loss alone. Studies show that many people stop taking their medications within three years due to side effects. Don, a fishing buddy of mine, showed up at the dock one morning with a face grotesquely swollen, which he thought was due to a something he ate. It was actually a reaction to the ACE inhibitor he had been taking for three years. The body can compensate for extended periods until it revolts when it is artificially manipulated by a drug poisoning.

As I mentioned before, always look to the drugs you are taking when side effects occur even if you have been on them for years.

Do nutrients really work?

Nutrients really do work, but don't believe just me. There is a wealth of research substantiating the need for nutrients to combat heart disease and related conditions such as high blood pressure, elevated cholesterol, diabetes, and macular degeneration. This research, which began 25 years ago, has grown from a trickle to a raging river.

There is no longer any mystery about the effects of nutrients. Science has shown, beyond any doubt, that the absence of proper nutrients is the cause of heart disease and related conditions. Harvard, Johns Hopkins, the National Institutes of Health, and nearly every major medical school have published articles showing the effectiveness of nutrients for prevention and treatment of heart disease.

The *New England Journal of Medicine*, *Journal of the American Medical Association*, and the *British Journal of Medicine* as well as many other respected peer reviewed journals around the world also have numerous articles highlighting studies that show spectacular results for the use of nutrients in prevention or reversal of heart disease. For example, research has shown that:

- Vitamin C, lysine, and proline (amino acids) act as Teflon agents to prevent further cholesterol build up.
- Lysine and proline are needed with vitamin C and the mineral copper to make collagen and elastin. Collagen strengthens arteries whereas elastin facilitates flexibility of the arteries.
- Arginine is an amino acid that can be turned into nitric oxide. In this form, it naturally relaxes arteries and reduces high blood pressure, prevents heart attacks, and repairs damage to arteries.
- Carnitine is a vitamin-like compound that increases the amount of blood pumped by the heart. It moves fat (fuel) into heart cells, decreases fat in the blood (triglycerides), improves heart function and increases the chance of survival after a heart attack.

- Coenzyme Q-10 increases the pumping efficiency of the heart muscle by 20 percent (more than any medication), and it has none of the side effects of heart medications.
- Folic acid, B-6 (pyridoxine), and B-12 (cyanocobalamin) are of supreme importance in protection against heart disease. These B vitamins prevent artery damage by reducing homocysteine in the blood. Homocysteine is a toxic byproduct of protein metabolism that damages arteries and causes heart disease. The processing of food depletes B vitamins. We are unable to combat the disease process stemming from B-vitamin deficiency without supplementation. Folic acid also decreases harmful homocysteine, which in turn, decreases the risk of heart disease. Lack of folic acid increases the risk of fatal coronary heart disease. Correspondingly, there is an increase in death rates in people with coronary artery disease due to folic acid deficiency.
- B-6 (pyridoxine) decreases an atherosclerotic buildup in arteries and prevents myocardial infarction (heart attack). B-6 and folic acid together decrease coronary artery disease in women.
- B-12 and folic acid reduce neural tube defects (spina bifida) and the risk of heart disease.
- Antioxidant vitamins A, C, and E prevent free radicals that cause damage to cells. This protection appears all the greater when we realize that cellular damage leads to cracking of the blood vessels, which leads to heart disease.
- Proanthocyanidins are very powerful plant antioxidants. Pycnogenol (from pine bark) is 20 to 50 times more potent than vitamins C and E in stopping

free radical damage. Proanthocyanidins from grape seed extract have been shown to lower cholesterol levels, prevent damage to the cell lining of the arteries, and shrink the size of cholesterol deposits in arteries.

- Phytonutrients have a powerful protective effect against heart disease by quenching free radicals.
- Chromium has been shown to lower bad cholesterol, raise good cholesterol, reduce insulin dysfunction (a major factor in heart disease), and prevent plaque formation.
- Selenium deficiency is the number one mineral associated with heart disease progression.
- Zinc is needed to reduce inflammation (a major cause of heart disease).

I'll discuss all of these vitamins and minerals in upcoming chapters.

Your doctor

If you don't agree with anything else I say in this book you should still replace the nutrients depleted from your body as a result of taking prescription drugs. Your doctor should advocate the same. The Hippocratic Oath states that a doctor should do no harm. If your doctor doesn't believe in or understand the value of nutrition—and let me tell you there are many who don't—I suggest you find yourself a more holistically-oriented doctor. I have nothing against conventional medical care, but I *am* against those who do not support replacing lost nutrients or taking nutrients to prevent and reverse heart disease.

5

Three Tests That Could Save Your Life

"A man is as old as his blood vessels."

> *— Sir William Osler (1849-1919)*
> *Considered one of the greatest physicians of all time*

As I discussed previously, standard risk factors for heart attack—high blood pressure, high cholesterol, being overweight and smoking—do not account for half of the heart attacks suffered. Then how do you know if you are at risk for heart disease? While the standard tests such as LDL (bad), HDL (good), total cholesterol, and triglycerides are important, there are three additional, newer tests that can really pick up heart attack risk. They are:

- C-reactive protein (hs-CRP).
- Homocysteine.
- Lipoprotein-a.

These tests will give you a more accurate assessment of your heart attack risk so you're ahead of the curve.

The government, medical establishment, and drug companies know about these tests, by the way, but say the tests are expensive and won't uncover more information than the standard tests. Nothing could be further from the truth. I encourage you to ask your doctor to run these on you.

C-reactive Protein (hs-CRP)

C-reactive protein (CRP) is a protein found in the blood. It appears in higher amounts when there is swelling or inflammation somewhere in your body.

Hs-CRP, which stand for "high sensitive C-reactive protein" is quickly becoming the mother of all tests. This is such an important test because science is showing that inflammation plays a much more important role in heart disease than was thought.

The older CRP test was a general marker for inflammation in the body, but the hs-CRP test can track inflammation to a more precise level.

According to the American Heart Association:

> Scientific studies have found that the higher the hs-CRP levels, the higher the risk of having a heart attack. In fact, the risk for heart attack in people in the upper third of hs-CRP levels has been determined to be twice that of those whose hs-CRP levels are in the lower third. These prospective studies include men, women and the elderly.

Knowing your high sensitive C-reactive protein levels can help you manage and lower your risk for heart disease. Anything over 3.0 mg/L (miligrams per liter) is high and the closer to 0 the better.

Homocysteine

Using elevated homocysteine levels as a risk factor for heart disease was popularized by Dr. Kilmer McCully in the

1980s. His work led to the homocysteine theory of heart disease. Studies indicated that people with high homocysteine levels had a greater incidence of heart attack or stroke. High levels of homocysteine are a better predictor of heart disease than all the cholesterol tests combined. People with high homocysteine and blocked coronary arteries have more strokes and heart attacks. You need to get your homocysteine levels down to 9 to 10 micromoles per liter (µmol/L0.

Lipoprotein (a)

LPa is a molecule that carries cholesterol through the blood. High levels increase the risk of heart attack. In fact, people can have no known risk factors and be at high risk of heart attack if their LPa is elevated.

A group of 100 cardiologists headed by Thomas A. Pearson, M.D., Ph.D., F.A.C.C., and Professor and Chair of the Department of Community and Preventive Medicine, reported on the case of a 57-year-old white male with no apparent cardiovascular risk factors. He did not have diabetes or high cholesterol and was a non-smoker. In addition, he was an active jogger and ate a nearly vegetarian diet. Even his homocysteine levels were normal. The only risk factor was a high LPa level. An angiogram revealed a 70 percent blockage in one of his coronary arteries.

The fun began when Dr. Pearson asked the other doctors to give treatment recommendations. All of the doctors recommended cholesterol-lowering drugs. Dr. Pearson reminded them that the patient's cholesterol levels were normal. He was trying to get them to recommend niacin, as this is part of the treatment to lower LPa. After they were reminded of the normal cholesterol numbers many of the doctors stayed with the cholesterol lowering drugs but were also willing to add niacin.[23]

High LPa levels can predict a heart attack when all other risk factors are absent. If your cholesterol numbers are good—and half the people who have heart attacks have normal cholesterol levels—it is a good idea to get your LPa levels checked. Less than 10 mg/dl (milligrams per deciliter) is good and anything over 25 is considered high. One of the ironies of having any of these three tests in an abnormal range is that they are responsive only to nutritional supplementation. High homocysteine responds to B-6, B-12, and folic acid. With elevated CRP carnitine, Coenzyme Q-10, vitamin C, vitamin D, and B vitamins are needed. And high LPa responds to all of the ingredients in high quality, balanced supplement, along with fish oils and added niacin.

Note: Fish oils must consist of EPA (eicosapentanoic acid), DHA (docosahexanoic acid), and GLA (gamma-linolenic acid) along with vitamin E to prevent oxidation (rancidity). Niacin should be taken in much larger doses than the RDA recommends, but there is the problem with flushing (a skin reaction to high niacin doses) and should only be taken under the supervision of a qualified physician.

6

The Amazing Aminos

"All those vitamins aren't to keep death at bay; they're to keep deterioration at bay."

– Jeanne Moreau
Actress

Amino acid therapy is a relatively new field. Amino acids are what proteins are made of, and are vital to human health. Ten years ago you couldn't find but a few articles on amino acids. Now there are thousands.

Over twenty years ago, the first amino acid to come on the scene, **Phenylalanine**, was highly touted by the holistic community, and many psychologists used it to treat depression. It worked well and some modest studies were done, but it fell by the wayside as most things do if they are not promoted by drug companies, the FDA, universities, and the media.

Arginine

One amino acid, in particular, has grabbed the headlines in recent years, but most people don't know its name: **Arginine**. Arginine produces a substance—nitric oxide—which is the active ingredient in Viagra. Nitric oxide improves sexual function by allowing blood vessels to dilate. You don't need to take Viagra, by the way, to experience its benefits. You just need to take 1000 milligrams of

Arginine—and you won't pay $5.00 a pill (which is about what Viagra costs).

In addition to improving sexual function, **Arginine can stop heart attacks, reduce plaque in your arteries, and lower blood pressure**. There are thousands of studies on Arginine and quite a few books devoted to its miracle properties. The book *No More Heart Disease* was written by Dr. Louis J. Ignaro, one of three doctors to receive the Noble Prize for his work on nitric oxide, which led to the development of Viagra and other similar drugs.

Research on Arginine

Let's look at some recent research studies about Arginine that are true eye openers.

- In 1996, University of Minnesota researchers published a paper in the journal *Circulation*, the official journal of the American Heart Association, showing patients with congestive heart failure to have improved circulation, increased walking distance, and an overall improvement in quality of life.

- In 1997, Dr. Rainer Boger and colleagues at the Hanover Medical School in Germany tested L-Arginine against Lovastatin, one of the major anti-statin (cholesterol lowering) drugs and found it far superior.

- In the 1997 August issue of *Circulation*, it was reported that Lovastatin had a weaker effect on plaque formation and artery wall thickening than L-Arginine.

- Researchers at the Medical College of Wisconsin found that L-Arginine was just as effective as vitamin E in stopping fat (LDL) oxidation and stopping free radical formation while the cholesterol-lowering drug Lovastatin increased free radicals.

- In 1997, the *Journal of the American Medical Association* reported that Arginine was shown to increase blood flow to the heart.
- The 1997, the *American Journal of Hypertension* found "Oral Arginine had beneficial effects on hypertension (high blood pressure)."

This is just a sampling of the current research on Arginine as a vital nutrient for cardiovascular health.

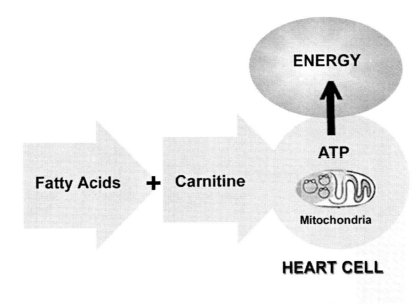

Carnitine

Cartinine is not actually a vitamin or amino acid. It's a protein-like substance that has vitamin properties. The reason why I talk about it in here is because it's made from a combination of two amino acids: **Lysine** and **Methionine**. Carnitine's major function is to transport fatty acids into the cells, especially the heart muscle cells, for use as fuel. So, Carnitine is a great benefit for heart disease.

The heart is the most important muscle and making sure its energy needs are met is paramount to long life. If you are over 35 you should be taking Carnitine as a preventative. If you have had a heart attack, it can protect your heart cells and stop any further damage that would lead to a second heart attack.

Carnitine and myocardial ischemia

Carnitine has also been shown to help myocardial ischemia (lack of blood supply to the heart). People with myocardial ischemia have plaque in their coronary arteries that reduces blood flow and decreases oxygen to heart muscle cells. This causes chest pain (angina) and irregular heartbeats (arrhythmias). Because Carnitine brings more fuel in the form of fatty acids to the mitochondria (manufacturing plant) inside the cells, oxygen to the cells increases.

This groundbreaking finding by Dr. Thomsen and Dr. Shug was published in the *American Journal of Cardiology* in 1979. Since then, eight newer studies have confirmed the results.

You may be confused by all the jargon or you may be thinking, "What does myocardial ischemia have to do with me?" The answer is simple: everyone is on their way to heart disease, so the sooner you start preventive measures the better.

Dr. Jack Strong M.D., chairman of the Louisiana State University Medical Center, reported in the 1999 *Journal of the American Medical Association* that plaque can build up as early as age 15. Although the onset of heart disease is gradual, you can have over 40 percent blockage without symptoms. Research even shows heart cells dying before symptoms occur. This is sobering to say the least.

More research

Carnitine has overwhelming evidence to supports its use for heart health. Still not convinced? Here a bigger sample of the increasing research on Carnitine.

- Dr. Carl Pepine M.D., professor and director of cardiology at University of Florida, published a study in *Clinical Therapeutics* in 1991 showing that improved exercise ability and better EKG results were obtained with Carnitine treatment.
- A 1995 *Journal of the American College of Clinical Cardiology* study showed that more heart muscle survived a heart attack when Carnitine was administered after the heart attack than the control group. It also prevented further damage.
- Another study in the *Post Graduate Medical Journal* confirmed the above results and further showed that the Carnitine group had smaller areas of heart muscle damage than those who did not receive Carnitine.
- Carnitine has been shown to improve nerve and vascular function in diabetics. [24]
- Finally, Carnitine lowers total cholesterol and increases (HDL) good cholesterol in diabetics.[25]

Synergism with Carnitine

Some synergistic combinations that increase health and decrease disease risk include:

- Carnitine, combined with vitamin C, naturally lowers cholesterol levels without harmful side effects of cholesterol-lowering medication.

- Carnitine, coupled with coenzyme Q-10, increases heart-pumping efficiency by 20 percent, more than any other treatment.

Cysteine

Cysteine is another important amino acid because it increases antioxidant formation and stops free radical damage to cells. It also eliminates toxic compounds from the body such as mercury. [26]

Lysine and Proline

If you do not have proper amounts of **Lysine** and **Proline**, you will not be able to form healthy collagen and strong elastic blood vessels.[27] Lysine and Proline act as a Teflon agent that prevents cholesterol from sticking to injured arteries. Without these two amino acids, blood vessels will become weak and crack under pressure, which starts the development of plaque in arteries leading to heart attack.

Collagen is the main component of connective tissue. It makes up about one third of our bodies. Our bodies make blood vessels, bone, cartilage and skin from collagen. When our bodies do not have enough vitamin C, they cannot use the amino acids Lysine and Proline to make the proper cross links in the collagen. All major disease processes spread because of their ability to eat through the collagen supporting structure and move to surrounding cells.

As with vitamin C, Lysine cannot be produced by the body. Our dietary intake is usually deficient in Lysine. Proline can be produced by the body but usually in inadequate quantities.

Dosage Range of amino acids: 50-200 mg per day.

7

Vitamin A

*"Vitamins are best taken in the correct
proportions to each other."*

— *Christiane Northrup, M.D.*
Physician and Author

Vitamin A, one of the four major anti oxidants in the body, is needed by the retina for both low light and color vision. Vitamin A also is vital for bone growth, reproduction, fighting infections, prevention of cataracts, the prevention of cancer in epithelial cells, and stroke and heart disease prevention.

Vitamin A was discovered in 1913 and is used to prevent night blindness (nyctalopia). Deficiency in vitamin A also causes drying of the membranes of the eyes (xerophthalmia). Xerophthalmia causes blindness in hundreds of thousands of children in developing countries, but is rare in the United States.

Excess vitamin A

Vitamin A is fat soluble and is stored in the liver. In rare cases, consuming excessive quantities of 200,000 IU a day can be toxic. Beta-carotene (pro-vitamin A), which is two molecules of vitamin A linked together, was discovered in

1932. Taking beta-carotene solves any potential toxicity problems. When the body needs vitamin A it just splits the bond holding vitamin A together. The body never converts more than it needs, so you won't have any excess.

Scientists believe that excess vitamin A inhibits vitamin D from allowing the body to absorb calcium. But without adequate calcium absorption, the bones get weaker and fracture more easily.

Adequate amounts of zinc are needed for the liver to release vitamin A for use in the body.

Research

Vitamin A has fallen out of favor due to a study linking vitamin A supplementation to an increased incidence of lung cancer. This study was done on 29,000 men in Europe who were heavy smokers and alcoholics for many years—a very sick group of people. Other research, however, shows vitamin A in a much more positive light:

- A 30 percent greater vitamin A dosage than the RDA recommends decreases the risk of breast cancer.[28]
- Vitamin A decreases heart attacks and strokes by 50 percent for people with existing cardiovascular disease.[29]
- Vitamin A decreases heart disease by 37 percent.[30]
- A Harvard study showed that vitamin A (beta carotene) reduces the risk of strokes by 69 percent.
- Vitamin A prevents cardiovascular disease.[31]
- Cancer rates were reduced with vitamins E, A, and selenium.[32]

Dietary deficiency

Although vitamin A deficiency that causes blindness is rare in the U.S., inadequate amounts in the diet can cause an increase in the risk of developing heart disease, stroke, and cancer. Taking supplements to insure against these conditions is a good idea as only 70 percent of beta carotene (pro vitamin A) is available from food while supplemental beta carotene is 100 percent converted to vitamin A.

Just getting the nutrient into the body does not solve all of the problems, however. Many say that you are just wasting your money on vitamins that end up in the toilet. This is not true if you have adequate absorption, transport, and storage in the body. You need to keep the supply high until tissue concentrations rise. This is like having a cup with holes in it; you have to keep overfilling the cup to overcome the loss from the holes.

In the case of older people who have lost some ability to absorb, transport, and store vitamins and minerals, the body must be supplied with excess to overcome this. This is solved by consistent nutrient intake.

All major studies show that supplements must be taken for two to five years to reach maximum benefit in disease prevention. That's one of the problems with vitamin deficiency—you don't feel sick until it's too late and you develop an active disease process. So, you need to start taking supplements now to prevent disease in the future.

Vitamin A

Some drawbacks with vitamin A have appeared in recent years. The most notable is that the dose of vitamin A that has shown benefits is a lot less than previously thought. We now know that too much, as well as too little, can increase the risk of hip fracture in older patients.[33]

It appears that 5,000 units are optimal. The research that supported higher doses was not solid enough to warrant a higher concentration.

Dosage Range: 2000-5000 iu per day.

Note: Milligrams and micrograms are self explanatory but sometimes vitamins are given in international units (iu) like vitamins A, D and E which are fat soluble. They are not exact equivalents in milligrams or micrograms but the biological activity they have in the body. The biological activity of one iu of vitamin A is equivalent to .341 of a microgram, forty iu of vitamin D to one microgram and 1 iu of vitamin E as D-Alpha Tocopheral succinate to .861 of a milligram.

8

B Healthy

*"Over 200,000 birth defects occur every year
in 80 countries due to inadequate B-vitamin
consumption."*

*— World Health Organization
2005*

The B vitamins are a group of eight vitamins and were once thought to be a single vitamin. Supplements containing all eight are generally referred to as a **vitamin B complex**. Individual B vitamins are referred to by their specific names (B-1, B-2, B-3, B-5, B-6, B-7, B-9, and B-12).

Just about everyone knows that you need B vitamins; they are beneficial and help the body in so many ways such as:

- Stopping cholesterol oxidation.
- Reducing plaque in arteries.
- Preventing Alzheimer's disease.
- Decreasing bone fractures.
- Preventing osteoporosis.
- Producing melatonin for proper sleep.
- Producing serotonin for proper nerve transmission.

Not getting enough B vitamins—especially B-1, B-2, B-3, B-6, folic acid and B-12—can cause many health problems.

The World Health Organization lists B vitamin deficiency as a major cause of health problems in impoverished nations.

Most B vitamins are water soluble and excreted in the urine, so you must take them daily to prevent deficiency.

So let's go through the B's so you can "b" healthy.

Vitamin B-1 (thiamine)

Vitamin B-1 (thiamine) deficiency causes Beriberi, a common malady discovered in 1920s in parts of Asia where the diet consists mainly of polished white rice. Beriberi causes severe neurological symptoms and even death.

Manufacturers used to polish rice by removing the husk, which contained the vital B vitamin, so the rice would last longer and not spoil in transit. Since then, laws have been enacted to require many foods to be fortified with B vitamins to prevent this and other diseases.

Government statistics show that over 45 percent of the American population is deficient in thiamine. Not only are many deficient to start with, but those who take diuretics for high blood pressure are even worse off as all diuretics cause thiamine as well as other B vitamin deficiencies.

If low levels of thiamine persist in the body it can lead to memory loss, depression, irritability, heart palpitations, pins and needles, and numbness. Dosage Range: 10-20 mg per day.

B-2 (riboflavin)

B-2 (riboflavin) deficiency can lead to Chelosis, which causes cracks in the corner of the mouth, inflamed lips and tongue, reddened, burning and itching eyes, excessive tears, and dry and itching skin. The U.S. Department of Agriculture estimates that 34 percent of Americans don't get enough riboflavin in their diet. Dosage Range: 2-15 mg per day.

B-3 (niacin)

Vitamin B-3 (niacin) deficiency causes Pellagra, a disease that causes the "three Ds" (dermatitis, diarrhea, and dementia). Pellagra is seen in countries where diets consist of mostly corn. Corn prevents the absorption of niacin. In Mexico, traditionally they treated the corn with alkali before eating it. This was thought to be unimportant until scientists found that the alkali increased niacin absorption.

B-3 (Niacin) is very important in reducing elevated cholesterol levels. In fact, if statins don't lower your cholesterol levels your doctor puts you on prescription niacin.

Niacin is also the treatment for lipoprotein-a which, when elevated, increases your risk of heart attack by 300 percent.[34] When you add chromium with niacin you double the cholesterol lowering effect of niacin alone.[35] This highlights the importance of taking a synergistically balanced formula that maximizes benefit. Dosage range: 15-2000 mg per day.

Have you ever had a sore on your tongue or inside your mouth that wasn't a canker sore? That's a mild form of Chelosis, a B-2 (Riboflavin) vitamin deficiency disease. The next time that happens, take three tablets of a B-vitamin complex, and in about two to four hours the soreness will go away like magic.

B-5 (pantothenic acid)

B-5 plays an important role in making hormones and neurotransmitters. Most people are not deficient, but you should take B-5 along with the other B vitamins to prevent imbalance. Dosage Range: 20-100 mg per day.

Vitamin B-6 (pyridoxine)

Vitamin B-6, or pyridoxine, deficiency can produce a torrent of symptoms such as nerve inflammation, PMS, skin problems and sleep disorders. Most people have heard the word "serotonin" but don't know exactly what it does. It's a neurotransmitter needed for proper sleep. If you don't get proper rest, everything in the body goes haywire. Psychiatrists tell us that you only need to lose two days of sleep before going into an altered state of consciousness. Anyone who has experienced the joys of a newborn can attest to that fact!

Most people know that you get sleepy after eating a turkey dinner due to tryptophan. That ties in with B-6 as it converts the tryptophan into serotonin. Without serotonin your goose (or turkey) is cooked. You'll never get proper rest.

Caution: Taking B-6 in very high doses can lead to neurological toxicity. Several studies have shown that if you take two grams tingling in hands and feet, stumbling, and decreased coordination occur. When the vitamin was discontinued, however, the symptoms disappeared. Dosage range: 10-100 mg per day.

B-7 (biotin)

Biotin is necessary for cell growth, the production of fatty acids and amino acids, and the metabolism of fats.

Recent studies have shown that biotin is essential in normalizing blood sugar and improving sugar metabolism in Type II diabetics.[36] Biotin is needed for proper hair and nail growth. Deficiency isn't common but could lead to skin rash, hair loss, high cholesterol and heart problems. Dosage Range: 50-500 mg per day.

B-9 (folic acid)

B-9, or folic acid, is a great story of how modern science reduced a terrible birth defect in children that left them deformed (Spina Bifida) and, in some cases, born without a brain (Ancephaly).

Unfortunately, these conditions develop in the first two weeks of pregnancy when most women don't know they are pregnant, Taking prenatal vitamins after conception is already too late. All women who are capable of getting pregnant should take folic acid as a preventative measure.

Newer research has shown that taking folic acid for one year before pregnancy has the added benefit of reducing premature births by 50 percent. Because premature babies suffer higher rates of cerebral palsy, birth defects, mental retardation, and are prone to more heart disease and diabetes, this highlights the need for much earlier supplementation.

Even before these findings, the CDC (Center for Disease Control) issued many warnings about the need for folic acid supplementation to prevent birth defects.

In a recent study published in an article in the *Los Angeles Times*, medical doctors stated that they didn't know that the average woman wasn't getting enough folic acid from their diets. Often, medical doctors are deficient in nutrition information because it wasn't in their training. Dosage Range: 200-800 mcg per day.

B-12 (cobalamin)

Vitamin B-12 deficiency can lead to macrocytic anemia, which means the blood cells get big and don't carry oxygen like they're supposed to. You can get rid of the symptoms of macrocytic anemia by taking folic acid, but the disease rages on. This is why folic acid must be coupled with B-12 to prevent people from getting worse. B-12 deficiency requires a long time to develop since the body stores a three to five year supply in the liver.

B-12 is hard to absorb from the digestive tract because, as we get older, the stomach produces less intrinsic factor (a glycoprotein), which is needed to absorb B-12. If you don't produce enough intrinsic factor you absorb less than one percent of the B-12 you take.

But new research shows that if you take a supplement with B-12, over time, blood and tissues levels will increase no matter your age or digestive condition.

Due to our high animal protein diet, most Americans get enough B-12. However, due to lowered intrinsic factor in older people and depletion by some prescription drugs, it's a good idea to take it.

You should also know that many drugs deplete B-12, especially the new proton pump inhibitors for acid reflux such as Prilosec, Prevacid, Protonix, and Nexium.

You can take B-12 everyday and your stores will increase. You can take an expensive B-12 spray or "sublingual B-12," but I suggest taking the right supplement, or going to your doctor and getting a B-12 shot for about $7.00 that will last you six months. Dosage Range: 100-500 mcg per day.

Research

Research on B vitamins includes:

- In a 1998 Harvard study, the risk of heart disease was cut in half by taking just double the RDA (recommended daily allowances) of folic acid and B-6 (pyridoxine).[37]
- Researchers were startled by two recent studies published in 2004. One showed a decrease risk of osteoporosis and broken bones, especially hip fractures in the elderly.[38] The second study showed that high homocysteine levels—which are lowered by B-vitamin supplementation—were an indicator of increased fracture risk.[39]
- Another study conducted at the Harvard School of Public Health found that increased folate (folic acid) levels were associated with a decrease in hemorrhagic strokes in men.[40]
- A study showed that taking B-6, B-12, and folate reduced restenosis (arteries closing up) by 48 percent.[41]
- In a study published in the 2000 *American Journal of Hypertensio*, three B vitamins (folic acid, B-6, and B-12) reversed plaque progression[42] as seen on ultrasound measurements. Another similar study showed that these vitamins stopped plaque progression even when treatment of the traditional risk factors was not working.[43]
- An increase in homocysteine levels doubles the risk of Alzheimer's disease. Since 70 percent of dementia cases are Alzheimer's disease and there is no known treatment or way to reduce risk factors, taking B vitamins could save millions from this horrible condition.[44]

Homocysteine controversy

Since the 90s, there have been numerous studies to implicate homocysteine as a major culprit in heart disease. Homocysteine levels can be reduced by taking vitamin B-6, B-12, and folic acid. However, there has been a concentrated effort to tarnish homocysteine and the B vitamins that reduce it. Three recently published studies showed no effect on heart disease and stroke. The problem was that all the studies were on people who already had advanced disease. The first study was done on patients with heart disease or diabetes; the second on patients who already had heart attacks; the third on patients who had experienced a stroke. In the last study, the patients who had the highest initial homocysteine levels had the greater risk of a second stroke.

These are cases of shutting the barn door after the horse is out. But do not be confused. If you need a reason to take B vitamins, remember their function in preventing plaque formation, fractures, and osteoporosis.

Elevated homocysteine accounted for about 15 percent of the population's risk for Alzheimer's disease. That means that if homocysteine were entirely removed from the complicated risk equation, 15 percent of cases would be prevented.

Scientist don't really know the links between vascular disease and Alzheimer's disease, but they do know that people who suffer a stroke develop dementia soon after. With Alzheimer's disease, it's not the plaque in the brain, but the toxic cloud of inflammatory byproducts, especially high levels of homocysteine.

B vitamins

A hitch with B vitamins is that taking too much of one can require you to take up to 25 times of another to compensate. You must take the B vitamins in the right amount and in the proper ratio to each other so you don't cause more problems.

9

Vitamin C

*"A vitamin is a substance that makes you ill if
you don't eat it."*

— *Albert Szent-Györgyi de Nagyrápolt
Discoverer of vitamin C*

L ack of vitamin C was known to cause scurvy as far back as Roman times. Scurvy causes fatigue, bruising, frequent colds, and artery damage. Some historians have attributed scurvy as the cause of losing the crusades as soldiers died from lack of fresh fruit or vegetables.

Sailors on board British naval ships often contracted scurvy because they did not have fresh fruits or vegetables. They would initially bleed from their gums, internal organs, and joints, and eventually die. In the 1800s, Dr. James Lind found that giving sailors lime juice prevented scurvy. It took 40 years before the British navy required that lime juice be stocked on all naval ships. (This is where the term *limeys* came from.)

Vitamin C itself wasn't discovered until 1928, when Dr. Albert Szent-Gyorgyi, M.D., Ph.D., synthesized ascorbic acid (vitamin C) in his lab, which earned him the Nobel Prize for science.

Scurvy is rare in modern society but there are a few documented cases of people who eat junk food with little or no fruits or vegetables that have come down with varying degrees of scurvy that responded to vitamin C administration.

The primary antioxidant

What does vitamin C do in the body? Besides being essential for collagen formation, it is the primary antioxidant in the body. **Oxidation** is a natural process like a pipe rusting or the breakdown of your wiper blades on your car. When exposed to heat and oxygen almost everything starts to break down due to oxidation. In the body, free radicals are formed from the thousands of oxidation reactions causing havoc on cells.

Vitamin C neutralizes free radicals and stops the oxidation process. Vitamin C also is needed to form many neurotransmitters in the body such as serotonin, norepinephrine, thyroxine, and corticosteroids. Normal sleep is dependent on proper creation of these hormones. The highest concentrations of vitamin C are found in the brain where it battles the aging process, and in the adrenal glands where it combats stress.

In addition to being the main antioxidant in the body, vitamin C also:

- Decreases harmful LDL and increases good HDL cholesterol.
- Dissolves atherosclerotic plaque.
- Boosts immunity and combats stress.
- Lowers blood pressure.
- Reverses damage to cells (endothelial) lining the blood vessels.
- Lowers mortality (death rate).
- Reduces incidence of stroke.
- Improves diabetes (glucose).

- Stops macular degeneration when combined with other nutrients.
- Decreases heart disease.
- Decrease levels of lipoprotein-a.
- Detoxifies lead, mercury, cadmium, and nickel.
- Improves nitric oxide function.
- Reduces the duration and severity of the common cold.
- Increases the healing of scars, broken bones and burns.
- Reduces the frequency and intensity of bronchial spasms in asthmatics.

Truly a miracle vitamin, wouldn't you say?

Vitamin C and collagen

Vitamin C is such an important nutrient in overall health because, without it, you cannot form collagen, the primary component of blood vessels. Without collagen, the blood vessels will break down and cause a host of problems.

To form healthy collagen and maintain endothelial cell health, the body needs the right raw materials. Vitamin C must have the amino acids lysine, proline, and the mineral copper to form the cross links that gives collagen its supportive structure and flexibility.

Vitamin C and blood vessel health

As Dr. R. Michael Cessna D.C., DACBI—the head of the post graduate division of the Chiropractic Internist Program at Texas Chiropractic College—used to say, "You're only as healthy as your blood vessels." That's certainly true. If a blood vessel in your brain ruptures, you get a stroke. If a blood vessel that supplies your heart fills with plaque, you can suffer a heart attack.

Diabetic death comes not from blood sugar levels but the effects of diabetes on the blood vessels which:

- Damages the fine blood vessels in the eye, causing blindness.
- Damages the vessels in the kidney, causing kidney disease.
- Breaks the fine capillaries to the legs, causing abscess, gangrene, and amputation.

A 2009 study in the *Journal of Clinical Endocrinology and Metabolism* showed that vitamin C, taken with insulin in Type I diabetes, stopped damage to endothelial cells lining the arteries and oxidation from free radicals.[45] There is no doubt that vitamin C is important for diabetics and blood vessel health. When is the last time you heard a medical doctor telling his diabetic patients to take vitamin C with their insulin to stop damage to their blood vessels? Probably never.

Research

A book is really needed to do justice, but here is just a short list of studies showing the broad spectrum of benefits in taking vitamin C.

Stopping plaque formation

In 1957, Dr. C.G. Willis reported in the *Canadian Medical Journal* how he reversed arterial plaque with the administration of vitamin C to heart patients.[46] More recent research shows that, as the primary antioxidant in the body, vitamin C stops LDL (low density lipoprotein) from oxidizing and forming plaque by scavenging free radicals.[47]

Additionally, it stops white blood cells from adhering to damaged endothelial cells, which is the starting point in the atherosclerotic process.[48]

Keeping arteries open

A study was done to see if vitamin C was superior to a drug in dilating vessels prior to a bypass graft. One thing doctors do not want to happen while doing a bypass is for the artery to shut down and cause a heart attack, either before or during the operation, so they prep you with a drug to keep your arteries open. This study showed that vitamin C was superior at keeping arteries open.[49]

Lowering blood pressure

As far back as 1987, doctors knew that nutritional and lifestyle changes would normalize blood pressure but instead jumped on the drug bandwagon. Why? The reasoning at that time, and still today, is that patients would or will not alter their diets or lifestyle. They believe that people are just too lazy to take care of themselves and it's easier to take a drug.

In a study of nutritional changes without drugs, 39 percent of patients lowered their blood pressure and maintained it four years after starting the program.[50] In another study, patients with Type II diabetes who took just 500 milligrams of vitamin C daily for one month lowered their blood pressure and improved arterial stiffness.[51] In a study that lasted 10 years, those who had the lowest levels of vitamin C had an almost three times greater chance of stroke.[52]

Lowering cholesterol levels

In a small but interesting study, the administration of just 1000 milligrams of vitamin C for four weeks reduced cholesterol levels by 16 percent.[53] In a much larger study, high vitamin C levels are associated with higher HDL levels (good cholesterol) and lower LDL (bad cholesterol) levels.[54] These were the same results from another study showing an increase in HDL and a decrease in LDL and blood pressure.

Reducing heart disease

In a 2003 study that followed over 85,000 women for over ten years, there was a marked decrease in heart disease from supplementation of vitamin C.[55] This was not from fruits and vegetables but from supplementation.

Analyzing the data from nine different studies, researchers found that those who took 700 milligrams had a lower incidence of coronary heart disease than those who didn't.[56]

Lowering mortality rates

In a large study called the First National Health and Nutrition Examination Survey (NHANES I), vitamin C was shown to lower death rates (mortality) in men, even after the researchers adjusted the data for factors like cigarette smoking, education, race and disease history.[57] And, again, when over 11,000 people were studied, those with the lowest levels of vitamin C and E had higher death rates.[58]

Detoxifying the body

There is a lot of worry about our toxic environment. Some, like smokers, accumulate lead. Others, like children, still get lead from old peeling paint on houses built before lead paint was banned in 1997. In both cases, vitamin C comes to the rescue as it detoxifies lead in the body so it can be excreted by the kidneys. It also detoxifies mercury, cadmium, and nickel. Youths who had the highest serum ascorbic acid (vitamin C) had an 89 percent lower prevalence of elevated blood lead levels compared with youths in the lowest serum ascorbic levels.[59]

Another study divided participants into three groups. The first group took a placebo (sugar pill), the second group took 200 milligrams of vitamin C, and the third group took 1000 milligrams of Vitamin C. The placebo and the 200 milligrams groups showed no reduction, while the 1000 milligrams group experienced reduced blood lead levels. This is a case where dosage levels are critical. The 1000 milligrams dose is sixteen times the RDA and was the only effective dose.[60] Not only can Vitamin C reduce lead levels, it can also prevent absorption when ingested.

Decreasing blood clot formation

Blood can coagulate (clot) by hitting a plaque deposit or clot spontaneously because the blood flow is too slow. The clot is made up of fibrinogen, which holds it together and forms a scab. So, two things happen after injury: the blood coagulates and the fibrin in the blood forms the clot. If you have high coagulation potential and high fibrin levels, you are more susceptible to clot formation and a heart attack. Low levels of vitamin C are associated with high levels of chemicals in the body that inhibit fibrin and coagulation factors in the blood.[61] [62]

Two more early studies indicated that heart disease patients who took 2000 to 3000 milligrams of vitamin C a day for one to six weeks increased fibrino-lytic activity (eats up the clot forming fibrin) and reduced platelet adhesiveness (sticky blood cells).[63] [64]

Plaque reversal

In the 1950s, Dr. C. G. Willis found that plaque in arteries could be reversed with vitamin C. Willis was a pioneer in the treatment of coronary artery disease. His work was ignored by the medical establishment and the fledgling drug companies. There was no profit in treating with vitamin C then, and it is still largely ignored today. Here, again, is a case of supplementation working far better than any drug treatment.

The following three photos show the reversal of atherosclerotic plaque from the artery of a guinea pig administered vitamin C. These photos, and the results of Dr. Willis' studies, can be found in the archives of the *Canadian Medical Journal*.[65]

This first photo is of atherosclerotic plaque build-up in the artery of a guinea pig that was deprived of vitamin C and shows the subsequent plaque buildup in the lining of the artery.

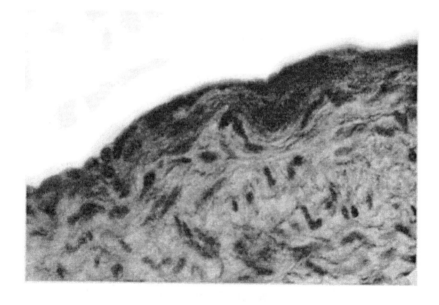

This next photo shows the reduction in plaque on the inside lining of the blood vessels.

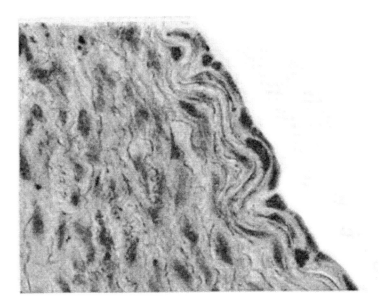

The last and most startling photo is the smooth artery lining absent any plaque formation after vitamin C was administered.

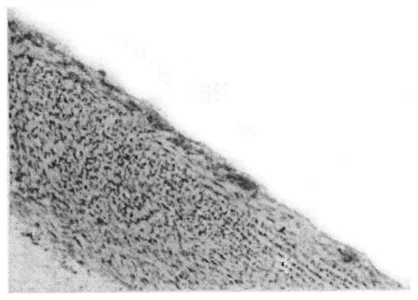

In 1996, a one-year study[66] was conducted on 55 patients with different degrees of coronary artery disease. The patients served as their own control group. Without the supplement program, the plaque buildup increased by 44 percent a year. So, without supplementation the deposits increase by half each year.

The following photo is of a patient that shows a reversal of deposits, or plaque, in the coronary arteries. The nutrient

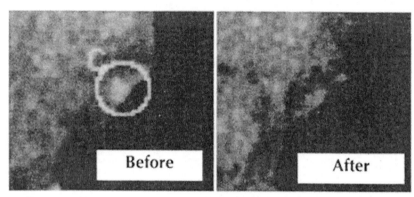

formula addresses the nutrient deficiency starting with the sub-clinical scurvy due to lack of vitamin C and the amino acids lysine and proline to form collagen. The photo on the left shows a blocked coronary artery and the one on the right show the reversal of the plaque in the same coronary artery.

Synergism

Vitamin C works in cooperation with many other nutrients.

- Vitamin C increases the effectiveness of vitamin E by recycling it 20 to 40 times. The body is truly a natural green machine.
- Vitamins A, C, E, and zinc purge the body of free radicals by forming antioxidants.

- Vitamin C, when combined with chromium, reduces cholesterol.
- Vitamin C, lysine, proline, and copper form collagen, which comprises 30 percent of the body.
- Vitamins A, C, E, zinc, and copper reduce the occurrence of macular degeneration (I talk about this in detail in Chapter 10).
- Coenzyme Q-10 needs vitamin C to be produced by the body.
- Folic acid needs vitamin C for proper assimilation and function in the body.

Vitamin C depletion

Depletion of vitamin C can be attributed to a number of reasons including stress and illness, drugs, and diet. Stressful situations (both physical and emotional) and severe illnesses tend to deplete the body's stores of vitamin C quickly.

There are three drugs that deplete vitamin C, two of which many people take on a daily basis: aspirin and birth control pills. The third is a class of drugs called loop diuretics that many heart patients are on. They include:

- Furosemide (Lasix).
- Bumetanide (Bumex).
- Ethacrynic acid (Edecrin).
- Choline magnesium.
- Trisalicylate.
- Corticosteroids.
- Ethacrynic acid.
- Torsemide.

Vitamin C deficiencies are found in elderly people on poor diets. Some studies have shown up to 95 percent of institutionalized elderly and 20 percent of healthy elderly are deficient. Seventy-five percent of cancer patients are deficient.

How much vitamin C is enough?

Initially, the recommended daily allowance (RDA) for vitamin C was 65 milligrams and was then increased to 75 milligrams. Scientists suggested that it be raised again to 200 milligrams due to the overwhelming research that supports its benefits. Current research shows 1000 milligrams to be the minimum daily requirement to prevent heart disease and numerous other conditions.

Humans do not produce any vitamin C, so they must get it from their diet or supplements. The body's vitamin C requirement is much higher than the RDA because it needs enough for construction of and repair to vessel walls, and to neutralize free radicals. The constant assault on the cells of the body from toxins and the byproducts of metabolism require more and more vitamin C. You have to keep filling the body with adequate amounts of C to overcome loss due to stress, toxins, and metabolic pollution.

When inadequate vitamin C is present in the blood plasma, it's replaced by lipoprotein-a in the artery wall and starts the plaque process.

Since vitamin C is water soluble you need to take it every day.

Vitamin C Types

There are four types of vitamin C:

- Ascorbic acid

- Calcium ascorbate
- Magnesium ascorbate
- Ascorbyl palmitate

There is no difference between ascorbic acid and natural vitamin C as they are the same chemical structure. Some advertisers would have you believe that there is a great risk of stomach irritation with vitamin C and say ester C is superior. Studies have shown ester C to be no better absorbed or utilized, so most that use it are simply paying more for good marketing.

Calcium and magnesium ascorbate are buffered forms of vitamin C and do not cause stomach irritation. I have treated thousands with these mineral ascorbates and have not had anyone complain.

The fourth vitamin C type is fat soluble ascorbyl palmitate, which is stored inside the cell membrane. It's superior at stopping fat (LDL) from oxidizing and preventing plaque buildup in the arteries. It's a potent ally in vascular health. Ascorbyl palmitate is missing from many formulas and shouldn't be.

Further reading

There is so much information on vitamin C that whole books have been written about it. In 1971, Dr. Irving Stone wrote *The Healing Factor: Vitamin C Against Disease*, which chronicles over 500 studies on the beneficial effects of vitamin C on numerous diseases. He was the force behind two-time Nobel Prize winner Dr. Linus Pauling's book, *Vitamin C and the Common Cold*, and his research into the effects of vitamin C in the 1970s. Dr. Pauling became quite a celebrity and started the vitamin C movement. He postulated that it would not only cure heart disease but cancer and the common cold. A good new book *Vitamin C: The Real Story* combines old and new research on the miraculous benefits of vitamin C therapy. Dosage Range: minimum 1000 mg per day preferably mixed ascorbic acid, mineral ascorbates and fat soluble forms.

10

Vitamin D

"Because vitamin D is so cheap and so clearly reduces all-cause mortality, I can say this with great certainty: Vitamin D represents the single most cost-effective medical intervention in the United States."

— Dr. Greg Plotnikoff
Medical Director, Penny George Institute
for Healing

Vitamin D is fast becoming a superstar in the vitamin world. Overlooked or thought to prevent only rickets in poor developing countries, it's now implicated in the reduction of breast, prostate, colon and pancreas cancer as well as heart disease and rheumatoid arthritis.

You can get vitamin D from food sources and from exposure to the sun. You need to get enough vitamin D in the summer to cover you during the winter. Many people, especially the elderly, stay indoors and do not get adequate stores built up. The older you get, the more your skin loses its ability to produce and manufacture vitamin D.

Vitamin D is a steroid vitamin that helps with the absorption and metabolism of calcium and phosphorous, which have various functions, especially the maintenance of healthy bones. Vitamin D is also an immune system regulator.

According to Dennis Bourdette, chairman of the Department of Neurology and director of the Multiple Sclerosis and Neuroimmunology Center at Oregon Health and Science University, vitamin D may reduce the risk of developing multiple sclerosis. Vitamin D is also linked to:

- Maintaining a healthy body weight.
- Reducing the frequency and severity of asthma symptoms.
- Reducing the risk of developing rheumatoid arthritis in women.

Despite vitamin D's health potential, about half of all adults and children are said to have less than optimum levels, and as many as 10 percent of children are highly deficient.[67]

Research

Research on vitamin D in the early 1990s showed benefits for reducing hip fractures and increasing bone density. Newer research shows benefits from everything from cancer prevention to improving heart disease, rheumatoid arthritis, and diabetes. Vitamin D is thought to be a preventative in over **seventeen types of cancer** including ovarian, prostate, Hodgkin's and non-Hodgkin's lymphoma.

In a study of cancer rates in Europe, vitamin D supplementation **showed vast reductions in all types of cancer**. Researchers estimated that reductions in cancer by supplementation would decrease cancer rates for men by 17 percent and women by 20 percent, resulting in a 16 to 25 billion health care cost savings.[68]

Vitamin D and colon cancer

The same study in Europe also showed a 50 percent reduction in colon cancer. It does this by neutralizing lithocholic acid, a toxic carcinogen. Note, however, that researchers cautioned against increased calcium levels due to high vitamin D intake.[69] However, I think the pluses far outweigh the minuses.

Vitamin D and pancreas cancer

In a Northwestern University in Chicago and Harvard University study of over 125,000 people who took supplements, vitamin D was shown to reduce the risk of pancreas cancer by 50 percent. There are over 32,000 cases of pancreas cancer in the U.S., and 95 percent die within five years of diagnosis. The people who took 400 IU of vitamin D had a 43 percent lower risk, while those who took 150 IU per day reduced risk to only 22 percent.[70]

And more...

Not enough data for you? Here's more:

- A study showed increased vitamin D intake reduced the risk of prostate cancer in men with metabolic syndrome. It also concluded that low vitamin D levels were strongly related to increased colon cancer risk.[71]

- A study published in 2006 showed that vitamin D levels were associated with increased benefit to the cardiovascular and immune system. And diabetics had a reduced risk of death from heart disease, one of the major causes of death in diabetics. Vitamin D is beneficial in heart and kidney function, apparently by reducing inflammation.[72]

- A smaller study done in 2003, published in the *American Journal of Cardiology*, points out the importance of vitamin D in preventing the progression to congestive heart failure in heart disease patients.[73]

- Vitamin D has been shown to reduce C-reactive protein levels and thus inflammation associated with rheumatoid arthritis. Toxic metabolites cause pain, stiffness and damage to bone in rheumatoid arthritis. Vitamin D not only improved symptoms, but reduced bone loss and stopped inflammation and the destructive process of rheumatoid arthritis.[74] I wonder how many rheumatologists recommend vitamin D to their patients.

- Another 2002 study published in the *Monthly Journal of the Association of Physicians* showed that people with a certain gene type were more susceptible to inflammatory disorders, such as heart disease and diabetes. But, by supplementing with vitamin D, it stopped tissue damage and inflammation in these conditions.[75]

Vitamin D is now shown to reduce overall death rates by stopping cancer, heart disease, and diabetes—the three main killers in the industrialized world. Researchers said, "Intake of ordinary doses of vitamin D supplements seems to be associated with decreases in total mortality rates."

Dosage Range: 2000 to 4000 mg per day.

11

Vitamin E

"Vitamin E is needed to sustain life and advance health."

> — *Suzy Cohen, RPh*
> *Pharmacist and Syndicated Columnist*

Vitamin E exists in eight different fat-soluble forms found in nature. The main form found and used in the body and added to food products is Alpha tocopherol (or α-tocopherol). This form is what is generally referred to as vitamin E and is the one most people buy off the shelf. The other vitamin E forms have not been well researched and are not needed except in rare circumstances. However, new research is showing promise for other forms, such as gamma and delta tocopherol. But until the research is more convincing, I do not recommend a more expensive type of vitamin E with all sub fractions.

The name tocopherol is derived from the Greek words tocos, meaning childbirth, and pherein, meaning to bring forth. The name was coined to highlight its essential role in the reproduction of various animal species. The ending -ol identifies the substance as being an alcohol.

What it does

Vitamin E is a major antioxidant in the body and **the most important vitamin in preventing heart disease**. Vitamin E's main function is to prevent oxidation of polyunsaturated fatty acids. Vitamin E also:

- Stops the fat in the cell walls from oxidizing, becoming rancid, and starting plaque formation in the arteries.
- Stops blood cells from becoming sticky and adhering to vessel walls, causing plaque or clot formation.
- Stops the blood from clotting by thinning it. This is why surgeons always caution against taking vitamin E before surgery.

It's like having your own private security guard protecting each cell.

Conditions vitamin E treats include:

- Heart disease.
- Cancer.
- Stroke.
- Alzheimer's disease.
- High cholesterol.

Research and the truth (or not)

Many drug companies, hospitals, and even some doctors discredit vitamin E for preventing heart disease. Why? They, of course, want you to buy their drugs and have surgeries that, in my opinion, are of marginal value and limited benefit. Taking vitamin E is not nearly as lucrative as selling blood pressure and cholesterol lowering medication.

Research studies confirm that you should take vitamins E and C after 40 when the risk of a sudden fatal heart attack increases to 49 percent.

For example, a recent study published in the *Journal of the American Medical Association*[76] followed approximately 40,000 women for ten years to see if vitamin E, from diet or supplements, decreased risks of cardiovascular disease and cancer. The researchers concluded, "These data do not support recommending vitamin E supplementation for cardiovascular disease or cancer prevention among healthy women." What they failed to mention, however, was that the study found "For cardiovascular death there was a significant 24% reduction." I'd say that's significant, wouldn't you?

And what's really odd is that the vitamin was given only every other day. Huh. Go figure. But this is the pattern I see over and over again. Design a faulty study and report only the data they want you to know. It's almost as if they are saying, "To tell you the truth, we're going to lie to you."

Remember the vitamin A study in Europe I talked about in Chapter 7? That study also tested vitamin E. They gave the participants 50 IU of vitamin E (three times the RDA) and found that there were **32 percent fewer diagnoses of prostate cancer** and **41 percent fewer prostate cancer deaths** compared to men who did not receive it.[77]

Prostate cancer is the most common type of cancer for men in the United States. Most men who undergo conventional medical treatment for prostate cancer end up impotent and incontinent for years, if not permanently. Prevention is a must. Why not use natural therapy that is cheap and effective and does not cause more

> How long you take a supplement and what other synergistic vitamins and minerals are present to increase effectiveness are really important.

pain and suffering? Take your vitamin E no matter what the doctors or the TV tells you.

Need more proof? I don't want to bore you, but there are a slew of studies supporting Vitamin E for heart disease. Check these out.

- Vitamin E **decreases heart attacks by almost 50 percent** according to a Cambridge Heart Antioxidant Study (CHAOS).[78] This clinical trial strongly supports evidence that vitamin E in dosages greater than 100 IU per day reduces CHD events. When they added vitamin C, the risk reduction was increased to 53 percent. And when taking vitamin E for even longer the risk was further reduced to 63 percent.

- A Harvard study[79] showed that taking just 100 IU of vitamin E per day for two years can **decrease the risk of heart attack by 46 percent**.

- A 1993 study of 39,000 men[80] found that **the risk of heart disease was reduced by 37 percent** with as little as 100 IU of vitamin E per day for at least two years.

- The World Health Organization studied 16 European populations and found that people with low serum (blood) concentrations of Vitamin E were **at much greater risk of heart disease** than those with high blood pressure and elevated cholesterol.

- Inflammation is now considered a major component in heart disease. **The major indictor of inflammation, CRP (C-reactive protein), was reduced by 30 percent** with vitamin E supplementation. Study co-author, Dr. Sridevi Devaraj, said, "The research suggests that vitamin E could be an additional therapy on our quest to reduce (heart) disease."[81]

- A *Journal of Clinical Nutrition* study showed **lower death rates for male smokers** who took vitamin E.[82]

- A 1999 study presented at an American Academy of Neurology meeting showed a **person's risk of stroke is reduced by 53 percent** if he or she takes a vitamin E supplement each day.

- Two studies showed that high levels of vitamin E led to a decrease in mental decline and a 70 percent reduction in the risk of developing Alzheimer's disease.[83]

These studies are just a few of hundreds done that show vitamin E to be a very important nutrient.

Deficiency in diet

Do we get enough vitamin E from our diet? The answer is no. The lack of proper amounts of vitamin E in our diets, along with loss from unsaturated fats or trans fats, leaves us exposed to heart disease. A John Hopkins study[84] showed that over one third of all Americans and 50 percent of African Americans were deficient in vitamin E. And those with the lowest concentration had the highest cholesterol levels.

The benefits of vitamin E can be dramatic when increasing your intake to 100 IU. And when increasing it from 200 to 400 IU, you achieve even better results such as a 50 percent decrease in heart attacks.

You may be interested to know that prior to the 1940s, heart disease was a rare condition. So what happened?

Milling processing methods invented in the 40s, and still used today, strip vitamin E from flour by taking the husk (wheat germ) from the wheat. The husk is the part that contains all of the essential vitamins and minerals. Vitamin E is also destroyed by heat and oxidation during cooking.

So, the average diet now contains only 30 IU of vitamin E. To get the amount necessary (400 IU) for optimum heart health from your diet, you would have to eat six cups of corn oil, 10 cups of peanut butter, or 100 cups of spinach.

Junk food and vitamin E

How about junk food? Well, you know it's not good for you, right? But it's hard to give it up. Just understand that after a high fat meal your blood levels of fat rise, the lining of the arteries becomes damaged, and your arteries go into spasm. Some research suggests heart attacks are exactly these kinds of spasms.

A patient of mine is a professional musician in Los Angeles who, after a gig, often goes to a fast food restaurant and gulps down a cheeseburger and fries. His buddies tell him he's killing himself. His reply is, "I'll be alright. I took my vitamins."

> When you eat fast food it reduces vitamin E intake. Fast foods have low levels of selenium and high levels of polyunsaturated fatty acids, both of which cause vitamin E depletion.

Can you really eat junk food and take vitamins and be fine? A recent study[85] seems to say yes. In that study, 20 healthy people were given 1,000 milligrams of vitamin C and 800 IU of vitamin E right before eating a high fat (50 grams) meal. The vitamins blocked or reduced vasoconstriction for six hours.

So, if you take the right supplement tablets before you eat a fast food meal you should be okay. I know, it seems ridiculous and it's not good medical advice, but the reality is that fast food has become an integral part of our lives. When the food supply is devoid of the proper nutrients, the only smart thing to do is to take the right vitamins along with the food. Why not? It works. The combination of nutrients in the tablets stops the damage to the artery wall and prevents spasm. That's good news for you Big Mac® lovers.

Natural versus synthetic

Many vitamins are not any different in synthetic form versus natural form, but this is not the case with vitamin E. The natural or d-α-tocopherol form of vitamin E is better than the synthetic form and is twice as effective. Various studies report that natural vitamin E has from 34 to 50 percent greater bioavailability (absorption) than the synthetic form.

An impressive case

So, the research makes an impressive case for vitamin E as an essential nutrient for heart health and disease prevention.

Additionally, vitamin C recycles vitamin E 20 to 50 times, so you don't need more than 200 IU. Remember, just as it is important not to take too little of a vitamin, it's also important not to take too much. Research from the 1980s about mega doses did not come back favorably. The Recommended Daily Allowance (RDA)—now the % Daily Value—is still woefully inadequate, but some of the earlier recommended high

> Vitamin E, when combined C and selenium, reduces the risk of cancer. Additionally, the body must maintain proper amounts of selenium to maintain vitamin E levels in the body.

doses did not prove to be correct. Dosage Range: 200-600 iu per day.

12

Chromium

"Chromium is critical in the metabolism of glucose and the action of insulin, but studies show that 90 percent of the American population has a chromium deficiency."

> *– Ray D. Strand*
> *Author, "What Your Doctor Doesn't Know About Nutritional Medicine May Be Killing You"*

C hromium is a trace mineral, which means that it's needed in very small quantities (micrograms instead of milligrams). Even though chromium was known about 200 years ago, it was not until 1929 that it was discovered. In 1959, Dr. Walter Mertz of the National Institutes of Health identified chromium as an essential trace mineral. Of the sixteen trace minerals, chromium is critical in insulin metabolism and blood sugar regulation.

Conditions chromium treats include hypercholesterolemia (high blood cholesterol), Type II diabetes, heart disease, and hypertriglyceridemia (elevated triglyceride levels).

Chromium's function and structure

The trivalent form of chromium is essential for the body and glucose metabolism. It's not the dangerous and disease causing hexavalent Chromium 6—the kind that's used to make bumpers and for chrome plating—exposed in the movie *Erin Brockovich*. Trivalent chromium, along with niacin, glycine, glutamic acid, and cysteine, is part of a complex called glucose tolerance factor (GTF), essential for proper sugar metabolism. Without this complex, the cells cannot absorb and use glucose.

This complex not only makes insulin more effective, thereby decreasing the risk of diabetes, it lowers cholesterol and triglycerides. People with high insulin levels are predisposed to diabetes and heart disease.[86] It's important to keep insulin levels in check with chromium supplementation.

Research

Let's start with some research articles on chromium. The first few are a little older, which I don't usually like to use, but they are still very interesting on the broad effects that chromium has on many health conditions.

- A study published in the *Western Journal of Medicine* in 1990[87] showed that taking chromium lowered bad blood cholesterol (LDL) and raised good (HDL) levels.
- Another small study done at Wayne State University in Detroit, Michigan showed that when niacin was combined with chromium, there was a 30 percent reduction in blood cholesterol levels.[88]
- An article in *Diabetes Obesity & Metabolism* cited a study that showed significant weight loss in women taking niacin bound chromium.[89]
- At Auburn University, Robert Lefavi, Ph.D. found that simply adding a niacin-bound chromium supplement to people's diets significantly lowered serum cholesterol by an average of 14 percent. This translates into a 28 percent decrease in heart attack risk. Additionally, the ratio of protective high-density lipoproteins (HDL) to total cholesterol, an important indicator of cardiac risk, improved by seven percent.

- Chromium was found to prevent plaque formation and stop cholesterol elevation.[90]
- Chromium supplementation resulted in a ten percent decrease in total cholesterol and a 14 percent increase in the good HDL cholesterol.[91]
- A study showed that taking chromium increased good HDL cholesterol and lowered insulin levels.[92]

Synergism: Chromium and grape seed extract

In 2000, the *Journal of Medicine* cited a study done at Georgetown University Medical Center, Washington, D.C. showing chromium lowered LDL. When grape seed extract, which contains proanthocyanadins (powerful anti-oxidants) was added, significantly greater reduction in blood cholesterol levels were achieved.[93] This is a prime example of synergism at work.

The researchers who studied the grape seed extract-chromium combination stated that the reason for doing the study was to find a natural way to lower cholesterol because there were too many serious side effects associated with cholesterol lowering drug treatment. This study, by the way, was done in the nutrition and physiology departments so they were not burdened by drug company involvement.

Chromium and diabetes

Another interesting study done in India, and published in *Biol Trace Elem Res* in 2004, noted people in the hospital who had to be fed by a feeding tube developed symptoms similar to diabetes. They gave the test group chromium and zinc, which seemed to solve the insulin malfunction causing diabetic symptoms.

Could nutrient deficiency be the cause of the diabetes? Another study done at Tel-Aviv University and published *Vitam*

Nutr Res in May of 2004[94] concluded that in a population of elderly diabetic patients undergoing rehabilitation, dietary supplementation with chromium was beneficial in moderating glucose intolerance. In addition, chromium intake appeared to lower plasma lipid levels. [95]

Chromium and dietary deficiency

Surveys suggest that over 90 percent of American diets are chromium deficient. Even when chromium is present in the soil, the plant form is poorly absorbed and utilized in the body. As you age, your body's level of chromium decreases. Chromium deficiency causes elevated blood sugar, numbness and tingling in extremities, nerve disorders in the limbs, and glucose intolerance.

Most people don't even know that they are chromium deficient, but with today's processed food diet it's really hard to avoid it. Here's the reason why. When you consume sugar— and average American consumes over 200 pounds of sugar a year—your body secrets insulin to bring your blood sugar level back to normal. The problem is that the insulin also brings chromium into the blood with it. The kidneys filter out this chromium so everybody who eats sugar is potentially chromium deficient. Chromium deficiency has very similar symptoms to the Type II diabetes, which is running rampant in the U.S. population. Dosage Range: 400-800 mcg per day.

13

Zinc

*"Almost 90 percent of all people fail to meet
even the so-called RDA for zinc on most
days."*

— *Dharma Singh Khalsa, M.D.*
Author, "Brain Longevity"

O ver 300 enzyme systems in the body need zinc to function properly. Zinc aids in wound healing, vision preservation, increases immune response, and offers protection from free radical damage. Zinc also decreases duration of the common cold and helps diabetes, macular degeneration, osteoporosis, peptic ulcers, Alzheimer's disease, rheumatoid arthritis, cardiovascular disease, and prevents benign prostatic hypertrophy (BPH).

Zinc and macular degeneration

Age-related macular degeneration (AMD) is the leading cause of blindness in people older than 50. A common feature of AMD is the presence of yellow deposits called drusen in the retina. Millions of elderly Americans have these deposits without vision loss and don't even know they have the disease. But, as the number of drusen and their size increase, vision begins to be affected. This is usually a long, slow process, and is called "dry" AMD.

For reasons that researchers do not understand, the process of deterioration can suddenly enter a new phase, called "wet" AMD, in which new blood vessels grow into the retina, producing bleeding and vision loss. It's frightening because people can move from a slow degenerative process to blindness in three months to six months. This is what researchers are trying to stop.

An age-related macular disease study showed that a vitamin combination of A, C, E, and zinc was effective for the treatment of macular degeneration, reducing progression of the disorder by about 25 percent. Eyebrows rose as there was no known drug treatment for macular degeneration prior to this vitamin combination.[96]

If all six million Americans with the disease were to take the cocktail of supplements for five years, "about a quarter of a million people who would have developed vision loss won't." said Dr. Emily Chew of the eye institute, one of the leaders of the study.

Dr. Thomas Friberg of the Eye and Ear Institute at the University of Pittsburgh said, "Historically, when you detected macular degeneration, there was nothing you could do to prevent progression."

Zinc deficiency and thyroid function

Zinc deficiency leads to lowered thyroid function as the body cannot convert thyroid hormones to their active form causing dysfunction.[97] And, in animals, studies low serum zinc concentrations resulted from diets deficient in zinc.[98] Let me tell you, if your thyroid isn't functioning properly, you experience a host of symptoms such as fatigue, irritability, constipation, elevated cholesterol and hypertension.

Zinc Benefits

As you can see, zinc is critical to good health and most people are deficient.

To help prevent macular degeneration, the correct combination is 500 milligrams of vitamin C, 400 IU of vitamin E, 15 milligrams of beta carotene, 80 milligrams of zinc, and two milligrams of copper.

Many of my patients, by the way, have told me that after taking a well-balanced supplement with zinc, they experienced hair and nail growth, especially in women who have thin hair and brittle nails. This is because of the zinc (and selenium) that is needed for a critical pathway in thyroid hormone metabolism.

Most people are selenium and zinc deficient so supplementation is a must. I'll discuss selenium in the next chapter. Dosage Range: 10-80 mg per day.

14

Selenium

"Selenium is an essential ingredient in your body's antioxidant system."

— *Hyla Cass, M.D.*
Author, "Supplement Your Prescription"

S elenium was thought to be toxic until 1957, when Schwartz and Foltz identified it as essential for human health. The 1970s produced a great number of animal studies identifying selenium deficiency with increased cancer rates, heart disease, decreased immune function and increased aging. In the last decade, newer research has come to light.

Structure and function

Selenium is needed for the glutathione peroxidase enzyme system, the most important immune protection system in the body. Glutathione destroys the damage (free radicals) caused by harmful unsaturated fats. Selenium:

- Is able to detoxify heavy metals, mercury, and cadmium.
- Is needed for proper thyroid function by converting thyroid hormone to its active form.
- Makes vitamin E more effective by increasing its antioxidant activity.

Dietary deficiency/drug induced depletion

It's been found that:

- Steroid use depletes the body of selenium.[99]
- Areas with lower selenium levels in the soil have higher arthritis levels.
- Food processing destroys selenium (wheat bread has twice the amount of selenium as processed white bread).
- Areas with higher selenium levels in the soil have lower cancer rates.

Conditions treated

A 1996 study published in the *Journal of the American Medical Association* was designed to see if selenium supplementation was effective for melanoma (skin cancer). It was not, but the study found that many other cancers were reduced by up to 45 percent. They stopped the study based on humanitarian reasons to give all of the participants the benefits of selenium supplementation.[100] (If there are dramatic decreases in the number of a potentially fatal disease with a treatment, they stop a study so all the participants can benefit.)

Based on these studies, the government of Finland has adopted a national policy of supplementation. It's ironic that our government has not done the same.

Selenium supplementation also was found to reduce serious and fatal heart disease (Keshan's disease) in children in the Keshan province of China. This condition, cardiomyopathy, is rare in children but there was an alarmingly high number in this province, 110 cases per

100,000 children when the number should have been one or two.

Researchers found that the soil was deficient in selenium so they gave a selenium supplement to every child in the control. The first year, the cases went from 110 to 56, and the next year they were down to 32 cases. They stopped the study and gave selenium to all of the children.

Synergism

In terms of synergism:

- Selenium potentiates (enhances or increases the effect of) vitamin E.
- Vitamins A, C, E, and selenium work synergistically to prevent cancer.

Selenium Benefits

Selenium is so essential to the human body—from its anti-inflammatory properties to cancer and heart disease prevention—that taking selenium is a no-brainer. Especially since soils are deficient in selenium and food processing dooms us to even lower amounts in our diets. Supplementation is a must. Dosage Range: 50-200 mcg per day.

15

Copper

"I got cocky and I stopped taking my vitamins. It was an inconvenience to have a suitcase full of vitamins with me on the road. About two years ago, it caught up with me."

— *Mary Anne Mobley*
Actress

Copper is an essential trace mineral and antioxidant that is absorbed in the small intestine, travels to the liver, and then on to the blood. Copper is a component in the superoxide dismutase (SOD) pathway, which is one of the body's most important antioxidant enzymes.

Structure and function

Copper is needed:
- To produce thyroid hormones.
- For iron absorption (which is needed to form red blood cells).
- For healthy connective tissue, especially collagen. Collagen synthesis is responsible for strong bone, cartilage, skin, and tendon formation.
- To produce elastin, which provides elasticity to arteries, preventing cracking and subsequent plaque formation.

Copper deficiency

Some researchers have shown that copper deficiency is associated with elevated cholesterol and triglycerides and the development of atherosclerosis. Thus, copper deficiency may play a role in the risk of cardiovascular disease.

Other research suggests that copper deficiency in youth could lead to artery defects that manifest as aneurysms in older age. This may be the reason that so many have aortic aneurysms later in life.

Copper deficiency is also associated with emphysema.

Benefits

Research shows that copper:

- Improves heart function and quality of life for those with congestive heart failure.[101]
- Stops LDL cholesterol from being oxidized.[102]
- Is a major plasma antioxidant.[103]
- Has anti-inflammatory activity and helps some forms of arthritis (a double-blind study showed that wearing copper bracelets relieved arthritic pain in some individuals).

Good news for chocolate lovers. Chocolate reduces LDL oxidation (due to its high flavanoid and copper content), which is good for heart disease prevention, so enjoy!

Two cautions

Too much zinc can cause copper depletion, but high doses of zinc are needed to prevent macular degeneration. People who have Wilson's disease, which causes toxic copper accumulation in the liver and other organs, should not supplement with copper. Dosage range: 2-4 mg per day.

16

Coenzyme Q-10

"Facing you are rows of vitamins and supplements for increasing vitality, sexual vigor, mental activity, you name it. Many medical investigators dismiss these 'cures' as hype. But that denunciation may be based on bias rather than on solid scientific evidence"

— James Goodwin, M.D. and Dr. Michael Tangum, M.D., medical commentators

C oenzyme Q-10 almost became the biggest nutrient of all time because it proved to be very effective in the treatment of heart disease in a study conducted in 1958 by Professor Karl Folkers, a research scientist at drug giant Merck Pharmaceuticals. Merck decided to go with a new diuretic called Diuril instead, and sold the patent rights to coenzyme Q-10 to a Japanese company. Coenzyme Q-10 is currently the best selling treatment for heart disease in Japan.

The body can synthesize coenzyme Q-10, but not in sufficient quantities. Low levels of coenzyme Q-10 are associated with congestive heart failure, high blood pressure, angina, stroke, arrhythmias, and lack of energy.

In a cruel piece of irony, the abandonment of coenzyme Q-10 and the incessant zeal to push cholesterol lowering drugs has led to a threefold increase in congestive heart failure after cholesterol lowering drugs came on the market in 1988.[104] Cholesterol lowering drugs were first introduced in 1987, and from 1988 to 1999 there was a tripling of rates of congestive heart failure. Why? Cholesterol drugs (statins) rob the body of coenzyme Q-10, which is one of the most vital nutrients for heart muscle health. Coenzyme Q-10 also lowers blood pressure by 10 to 15 percent.[105]

As the following chart shows, cholesterol is in the same pathway that produces coenzyme Q-10. Cholesterol lowering drugs work by blocking HMG-CoA from producing Melvalonate, which stops cholesterol production, but also stops coenzyme Q-10 production, which is vital for heart cells. Anyone who takes a statin drug must supplement with Coenzyme Q-10.

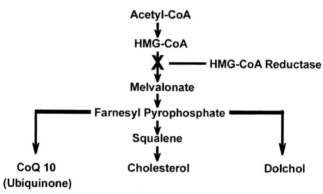

Benefits of coenzyme Q-10

Little known is the fact that coenzyme Q-10 regenerates vitamins C, E, and A, making it a potent antioxidant enhancer. It also stops oxidation of LDL (bad) cholesterol, increases HDL (good) cholesterol, and lowers blood pressure. Has your doctor told you about coenzyme Q-10? I'm betting not. Sadly, most doctors are too busy or were never educated about natural therapies' incredible success.

Coenzyme Q-10 Benefits

It's important to keep in mind that the production of coenzyme Q-10 is a 17-step process, which requires vitamins B-2, B-3, B-5, B-6, B-12, folic acid, and many trace elements. You can take coenzyme Q-10 but you should also give your body all the above nutrients to make your own. You don't want to take nutrition just like drugs. You need to take all the building blocks to produce your own. Not only does your body get coenzyme Q-10 it recognizes Co Q-10 and starts to produce its own. This is why you must take all of the nutrients together or you will be jeopardizing heart function by incomplete supplementation. Dosage range: 20-200 mg per day.

17

Pycnogenol, Proanthocynadins, and Bioflavonoids

"To all my little Hulkamaniacs, say your prayers, take your vitamins, and you will never go wrong."

— Hulk Hogan
Professional wrestler

Pycnogenol, from the Maritime Pine tree, is a phenomenal anti-inflammatory nutrient and is good in treating auto immune and cardiovascular disease. It stops the immune response that injures the artery, which starts the plaque process in cardiovascular disease. These are critical nutrients in the fight against heart disease.[106]

Pycnogenol and grape seed extract (proanthocyanidins) together protect vessel walls and prevent atherosclerosis. They also stop the inflammatory response in the body. Grape seed extract stops inflammation, scavenges free radicals, stops fats from oxidizing, and stops formation of inflammatory by-products.[107]

Pycnogenol, when taken with an ACE inhibitor, results in decreased blood pressure, protecting diabetics from kidney damage.[108]

Bioflavonoids are recently discovered plant compounds that have shown great success in protecting vessel walls and preventing atherosclerosis as well as many other conditions.

Research has shown that those with higher bioflavonoid content have lower death rates from heart disease.[109] Bioflavonoids also:

- Prevent free radical damage (by being an antioxidant that is 20 to 50 times more potent than vitamins C and E)
- Improve eye circulation in diabetes preventing retinopathy.[110]
- Improve venous insufficiency and retinal micro-hemorrhages.[111]
- Regenerate and protect vitamins C and E.[112]
- Improve lung function in asthmatics.

Dosage range: Pycnogenol (20-100 mg per day), proanthocyanadins-grape seed extract-(20-100 mg per day) and bioflavonoids (100-200 mg per day).

18

Glucosamine Sulfate and Lutein

"There's a new science out called orthomolecular medicine. You correct the chemical imbalance with amino acids and vitamins and minerals that are naturally in the body."

> — *Margot Kidder*
> *Actress*

Glucosamine sulfate is a glycoprotein needed for the formation of mucin, which is the coating on the intestinal wall. Glucosamine sulphate repairs the mucosal lining so that vitamins and nutrients can be absorbed into the blood stream.[113] It also rebuilds and repairs cartilage in the body. Glucosamine sulphate is excellent for arthritis, as it rebuilds the cartilage that is worn out and provides the body with sulfur (research has shown most arthritis sufferers are deficient in sulfur). Additionally, glucosamine sulfate decreases the incidence of kidney stones.

Glucosamine sulphate is far superior to conventional therapies, such as ibuprofen, which causes more joint damage the longer you use it (and is also the leading cause of kidney failure). Acetaminophen, the active ingredient in Tylenol, also causes kidney damage and is the number two reason for emergency room admissions in the United States.

Lutein, an antioxidant that protects the macula from light, is a member of the carotinoid family. Lutein delays the progression of macular degeneration, the number one cause of blindness in seniors.[114][115]. Lutein also decreases cataract formation,[116] slows progression of retinitis pigmentosa (progressive vision loss until blindness occurs),[117] and reduces eye inflammation leading to vision loss.[118]

Dosage Range: Glucosamine (200 mg per day), Lutein (20-100 mg per day.

19

The Rest of
the Gang

H ere's the rest of the gang, including calcium, magnesium, potassium, phosphorus, molybdenum, and inositol.

Calcium, along with Vitamin D (made via either supplements or sunshine), is needed to prevent rickets and to maintain proper bone formation. Signs of calcium deficiency include muscle cramps, high blood pressure, and heart palpitations. Studies have shown that calcium:

- Decreases osteoporosis and bone loss.[119]
- Reduces high blood pressure.[120]
- Lowers blood pressure in pregnant women.[121]
- Reduces both diastolic and systolic blood pressure.[122]

One reason we are calcium deficient is due to high-phosphorus foods such as soft drinks and too much animal protein. Additionally, lack of exercise, a low fiber diet, and too much fat consumption compound the problem. Our food supply is so deficient in proper mineral content that it is fair to say the most everyone is mineral deficient to some degree making supplementation a must.

When taking calcium, you need to take it with other nutrients rather than by itself. A study showed a two to three time increase in bone density when taken with other nutrients. This highlights my insistence on taking a complete formula for maximum synergistic benefit.

In fact, calcium, magnesium, sodium, and potassium should be taken together, as an excess of one can cause a deficiency of the other.

Magnesium

Magnesium is a very important mineral that is used in over 300 different biochemical reactions. A study of over 14,000 people over 15 years showed that people with low blood levels of magnesium had a 25 percent increased risk of stroke. Magnesium deficiency can also lead to artery spasms and sudden death.[123]

Supplementation is shown to be beneficial for heart function as it reduces disarrhythmias (irregular heartbeat) after cardiac surgery.[124] Magnesium also reduces high blood pressure.[125]

Oral supplementation with magnesium aspartate-HCl may lower blood pressure in subjects with mild to moderate hypertension.[126]

Lifestyle changes, along with adequate magnesium intake, can benefit blood pressure control, promote weight loss, and improve chronic disease risk.[127] (100 mg per day)

Potassium

Potassium is the most important electrolyte (electrical conductor). Potassium lowers blood pressure. It is of benefit in treating hypertension, especially when there has been a high intake of sodium. Authors of a 1999 study stated:

> "Increased potassium intake should be included as a recommendation for prevention and treatment of hypertension, especially in those who are unable to

reduce their intake of sodium. Other suggestions for reduction of blood pressure recommended by the authors are weight loss, reduction of sodium intake, moderation in alcohol consumption and increased physical activity."[128]

The authors of this study make clear that non pharmacologic treatment is important in controlling hypertension, especially for those who are salt sensitive or have a family history of hypertension. In fact, the longer potassium supplements were taken, the better the result.[129]

In another study, potassium had a blood pressure lowering effect in people with low dietary intake.[130] (50-200 mg per day)

Phosphorus

Phosphorus stimulates normal contraction of the heart muscle. And niacin (B-3) and riboflavin (B-2) cannot be digested unless phosphorus is present in the body. (no more than 1000 mg per day from all sources as there is too much phosphorus in the American diet)

Molybdenum

Molybdenum is present in every cell of the body, but only a small amount is needed for proper health. It's important in many enzyme systems in the body. Molybdenum detoxifies the body from sulfur-containing compounds, is important in anti-oxidant functions, and affects iron and copper absorption.

There is a common deficiency of Molybdenum in the general population.[131] (200-600 mcg per day)

Inositol

Inositol helps the liver remove excess fat from body tissues. It prevents fat buildup and inhibits tumor growth when combined with B-6 (pyridoxine).[132] It's effective in treating depression and is helpful in diabetic neuropathy. (50-100 mg per day)

20

Your Diet

"Don't dig your grave with your own knife and fork."

— English Proverb

All diets work—Atkins, South Beach, Weight Watchers, Jenny Craig, Carbohydrate Addicts Diet, The Zone, Eat Right for Your Blood Type, the Beverly Hills' Diet, Scarsdale, and a thousand others. Low fat, low carb, low calorie. They *all* work.

Anyone can change their habits for two to three months and lose 20 pounds. Inevitably, however, most of us revert to our old ways and regain the weight. And, to add insult to injury, we often add a few more pounds.

And even if you do maintain a diet for a time, most people fall off the wagon for either the slightest upset (holidays, bad mood, depression, rejection) or more severe events (divorce, a death in the family, lost job).

Good news/bad news

The good news is that Americans consume high amounts of protein, which is needed (especially as we age), although more fish and poultry would greatly benefit overall health.

The bad news is the Standard American (SAD) diet, which is high in refined, processed, synthetic, and superheated trans fats with an excess of sterilized salt, is a major problem. Eating these fats leads to oxidation and free radical damage.

As I mentioned in an earlier chapter, eating fast food gives you a load of these fats, but, if you take the correct antioxidants along with the occasional bad fats you will prevent artery damage. The best thing to do, however, is to stop eating trans fats.

It's easier to take a pill

Science shows that if you lock an overweight person in a padded room and give him or her only 2000 calories a day, he or she will lose weight. But drug and processed food manufacturers—as well as many consumers themselves—maintain that changing eating (and exercise) habits are too difficult, so don't bother—just take drugs if you get high blood pressure or high cholesterol.

Hints from centenarians

If you look at the diets and lifestyles of centenarians (people over 100 years old), you will see that there is a lot of hype about diet and exercise that is not true. There are over 60,000 centenarians in the U.S. and it's estimated that this number will rise to over 250,000 in the next twenty years.[133] Now, by and large, these folks didn't watch what they ate and there were certainly no gyms to work out in, as the fitness industry hadn't been born yet. The only thing that stands out was that they were, for the most part, never overweight. Data suggests that what you eat and how much you exercise has nothing to do with longevity.

Changing the paradigm

What, exactly, does it take to change your habits? What are the benefits? Is it painful? Can anyone do it? Can *I* do it? These are all great questions. To change your eating paradigm, you must be in a constant state of self-awareness and vigilance.

It's the analogy of a garden. You prepare the soil, plant, water, feed, and prune the plants. You get it just right. You enjoy the beautiful colors and fragrances and pluck the weeds as they pop up. But if you forget to tend the garden regularly, or just don't feel like it, those nasty weeds invade and take over. If you give up completely, your garden will turn into a wild heap of out-of-control nature.

Knowledge is key. You must know that food is actually your body's medicine. You need to learn about what you should be eating and what nutrients to take and why.

Let's look at the various diets and other good and bad foods.

The low fat diet myth

The low fat diet is one of the most prevalent and phony myths promoted to the American public. There is no scientific evidence showing a low fat diet to be healthful. In many cases it is detrimental to health.

A March 2001 *British Medical Journal* article showed that fat had little effect on cardiovascular disease in over 40 studies. A major study published the *Journal of the American Medical Association* in 2006 showed that a low fat diet did not lower breast cancer, colon cancer, and heart disease rates.[134] And, a January 13, 2010 online article published by the *American Journal of Clinical Nutrition* showed no correlation with heart attacks to fat consumption when analyzing over 21 studies with over 348,000 adults.

This puts a major monkey wrench on the low fat diet craze. If the media gives up on cholesterol as the cause of heart disease, both the low fat food manufactures and the drug companies that make cholesterol-lowering drugs would collapse and they'd lose billions.

High carb diets

High carb diets cause the body to secrete too much insulin because carbs are quickly broken down into sugar. You can't pour in sugar and secrete tons of insulin. Why?

- The insulin will become ineffective.
- The body will produce inferior insulin.
- The cells will not respond to the insulin.
- The body will store the sugar as fat.

This excess insulin lowers the blood sugar too much and the body becomes hypoglycemic (low blood sugar), which triggers more eating. This vicious cycle leads to weight gain, Type II diabetes, and heart disease.

Eat less refined carbs, very little sugar, and more complex carbohydrates with low glycemic index—the number that tells how quickly the body turns a food into sugar. The quicker your body turns it into sugar, the faster it disrupts normal metabolism. Even eating pasta cooked al dente (firm), and not cooking it to mush, has a lower glycemic index as it's turned into sugar slower.

The high protein, low carb diet did not originate with Dr. Atkins, but from a study in the1950s that showed low or no carbs and high protein caused overweight subjects to lose weight. There are always critics of new successful diets, but the problem with the Atkins diet is that too much protein is not good because it puts too much stress on the kidneys and causes bone loss to buffer the excess acidity. But eating only vegetables and protein *will* make you lose weight.

The Mediterranean diet

If you take indigenous people from Hawaii or Okinawa, Japan and superimpose a typical American fast food diet—high in carbohydrates and refined and processed foods—you increase the incidence of all of the common ailments we suffer including diabetes, heart disease, and the like.

If you give people refined food devoid of vitamins and minerals, whether it is by soil depletion or processing, you will still have sick people.

The best diet for heart disease prevention is the Mediterranean diet, the diet of Southern Italy and Greece, which emphasizes antioxidant and omega-3 fatty acid foods. Half of the diet is carbohydrates, 20 percent is protein, and 30 is fat (predominately olive oil, which I consider to be one of nature's perfect foods). Most of the food is fresh and locally grown with minimal processing. It's really not a diet, but a cultural eating style.

And, I don't think it's that hard for Americans to follow because it's not far off from the diet you already eat. Here's an overview:

- Vegetables and fruits (five servings daily, full of vitamins C and E and antioxidants believed to reduce risk of neurological conditions like Alzheimer's disease).
- Good fats, mainly olive oil, known for its cholesterol-lowering, blood sugar-lowering, and inflammatory-fighting properties.
- Legumes (lima bean, lentils, navy beans, black beans and kidney beans).

- Nuts and seeds (such as, a daily handful of walnuts, almonds, hazel nuts or pecans, which are low in saturated fat).
- Whole-grain bread, pasta, and potatoes.
- Milk and dairy, moderate consumption.
- Fish (a few times a week).
- Poultry and other lean meats and no (or little) red meat.
- A glass of wine or two a day (this is the best part of the diet, but I don't recommend alcohol consumption; grape juice will do the same thing without the dangers of alcohol consumption).

This diet leads to a:
- Nine percent reduction in all mortality incidences.
- Nine percent reduction in cardiovascular disease risk[135]
- Six percent reduction in cancer risk.
- Thirteen percent reduction in Parkinson's and Alzheimer's risk.

A study done by Michel de Lorgeril at the Lyon Heart Study of the French national Institute of Health and published in *Circulation* in February 1999 showed that the Mediterranean diet resulted in a 70 percent reduction in heart attack compared to the Standard American diet (SAD). In addition, the benefits were not related to cholesterol levels. The problem is not cholesterol but dietary deficiency. In fact, Dr. Lorgeril believes that the diet's protective effect comes from omega-3 fatty acids, fresh fruits, vegetables, vitamins, minerals and bioflavonoids.[136]

The above results are superior to any drug regimen and have none of the side effects—and don't cost a dime more than you are already spending on food. In fact, the diet is cheaper as fruits, vegetables, and olive oil are rather reasonably priced and the savings on meat is an added bonus. Food is a much better medicine than drugs will ever be.

French paradox

If the Mediterranean diet is convincing enough, here comes the French paradox. The French eat a diet high in saturated fats and have low rates of heart disease. What gives? How could this be, as it flies in the face of our low fat religion in the U.S.

Some would say it's the fresh produce, but this does not explain why their increase in saturated fat consumption has lowered heart disease rates. Just another fly in the ointment for the low fat craze.

Iodine

Iodine is one of the main components of the Japanese and long-lived Asian diets. They get it from seaweed (Nori) and many other fermented foods. I recommend that you get natural sea salt, as the table salt we use is a sterile chemical concoction without adequate iodine and absent the 40 plus minerals in natural sea salt.

Iodine is essential for adequate thyroid function, which controls the metabolism of every cell in the body. Even mild subclinical thyroid dysfunction can lead to heart disease.

Fruit

Almost all studies show that eating fruit improves health, and half the studies show cancer prevention when eating three or more fruits a day. You must incorporate fruit into your diet. Try everything. There are many varieties of apples, new crispy pears, apricots, plums, and a host of other fruits. We are blessed with an abundance of fruit from around the world, so fresh fruit is available year round. Adopt a fruit. Find one you like and eat it—it's just that simple. Instead of chips,

A word of warning: there are toxins on fruit, so be sure to wash all fruit thoroughly (although this does not eliminate all pesticides, unfortunately).

cookies, or ice cream, have a delicious succulent piece of your favorite fruit. Eat organic fruit, if possible.

Low calorie consumption

One of the reasons that Okinawans, Vilcabambans, and Hunzakuts—three of the longest living peoples on the planet—live so long free of disease is that they have low calorie intake. In other words, most Americans overeat and dig their graves with their forks. In fact, calorie restriction has been the only proven scientific method to increase life span. In the 1980's, Dr. Roy Wolford, a scientist at UCLA, was the pioneer in this field. He showed that mice lived longer on calorie-restricted diets. More studies including monkeys have shown the same result.

Soy

Scientists are touting the effects of soy protein in the diet to reduce cancers and all sorts of disease. The problem is that they don't know if the results are due to people eating soy starting when they were kids or whether you can start eating soy when you're an adult and reap the benefits. Eating soy when you are older can cause cancer, as there are estrogen-like side effects from soy consumption. Don't take soy as a supplement in my opinion.

The rebound phenomenon

I mentioned earlier that the average person who goes on a diet ends up gaining back all of the pounds they lost, plus more. This happens because your body is responding to you starving it; it wants to make sure you have enough weight in case you do a crazy thing like that again.

This is called the rebound phenomenon and it happens with all diets. It even happens with exercise. At first you lose weight with an hour of aerobics, but as you continue, your body adjusts. Now the body will lower your metabolism and you will burn 600 calories instead of the 800 you were burning at the beginning. Interval training overcomes this problem. I'll talk about it more in the next chapter.

This double whammy is hard to overcome. Workout more and burn less calories, and as soon as you stop a diet the body adds extra weight. No wonder diets don't work.

Here's the thing. You need to make *permanent* eating changes to have any lasting effect and to overcome this starvation reaction and metabolism recalibration. Changing your habits is the only real way to lose weight.

How to change

The painful truth is that we are a country of overfed and undernourished gluttons. The media demonizes fat as the culprit making you feel guilty, but the real villain is gluttony. Scientific studies show that eating a 2000-calorie a day diet is sufficient to provide for the body's daily needs.

The good news is, there are four small changes that are easy to make but that really matter to your health. They include:

- Eat a vegetarian meal once a week.
- Eat fish once a week.
- Use olive oil.
- Eat nuts.

Veggie night

Just making one meal per week vegetarian will greatly improve your health. It won't kill you to have a salad and rice with vegetables, or a bean soup with a salad and whole wheat bread, or even pasta with a salad and vegetables. You will feel better, have more energy, and sleep better. It's very good to give your body a break from the animal protein eaten almost every night by Americans. Cut down, also, on the portion of your meat serving; three to four ounces is enough.

Fish night

Research shows that eating fish just once a week improves cardiac profile and reduces heart disease risk by 34 percent.

There is a danger with too much fish as they are polluted with high mercury content and many others toxins like PBC's, so limit your fish consumption to once or twice a week

Olive oil is your best friend

Researchers know that for every ten points your blood pressure goes up, your chance of heart attack increases by 46 percent. But a study published in 2000 in the *Archives of Internal Medicine*[137] show that taking olive oil led to an eight point drop in blood pressure and cut the need for medication by almost half. Olive oil is a must. Now olive oil is mainly omega-9 oil which is excellent for the body and a primary reason the Mediterranean diet works so well. It is not that we don't get enough omega-3 but we eat too much of the wrong kind of omega-6 (corn, safflower and sunflower) and certainly not enough of the omega-9 found in olive oil. Olive oil is so darn good. Slather it on everything, just as the Greeks and Italians do. Make your own salad dressing. Mix olive oil, a few tablespoons of vinegar, salt, pepper, and a little sugar to taste—and voila!

Be a nut

Nuts are excellent sources of fat (the good kind) and contain much-needed vitamins and minerals. Brazil nuts have some of the highest selenium content of any food because the soil they're grown in has high selenium content.

The toxic diet

Most people don't realize that they have a second diet: a toxic diet. We not only ingest toxins and chemicals from our food, but also from our environment by breathing, through skin absorption, and through the water we drink.

There are literally thousands of chemicals and pollutants that we consume each day—everything from PCB's to mercury, chlorine and fluoride, Teflon, TCE (trichloroethylene) from military waste, to toxic bromide-based flame retardant in TV's, cars, furniture, computers, and just about everything you could imagine. There is even a carcinogen 1,4-dioxane in shampoo and bath products. I am just scratching the surface. All of them lead to health problems, especially cancer and heart disease. Many are carcinogens and the others cause inflammation that cause heart disease. Avoid exposure at all costs.

The main problem is the accumulated dose. It's the analogy of a baseball player who doesn't have to hit a home run to score for his team. The bases could already be loaded and a single will score. Likewise, one more toxic dose—ingested by using pesticides on your lawn, or working a short time at a job that exposes you to toxins, or eating fruits and vegetables that are contaminated with pesticides, or even moving next to a major highway and inhaling toxic diesel exhaust—can be the single event that can cause cancer or heart disease.

One bright spot is that many nutrients such vitamin C and the mineral selenium can neutralize and eliminate toxins—including mercury, lead, and fluoride—from the body.

Relax. Things take time and habits are hard to break. Gradually start changing your diet and add vitamins and exercise. Limit your toxic exposure as much as possible. Reread the chapters on the nutrients and the research that shows their benefit. This will bolster your resolve and give you added encouragement. Continue to diet and, if you fail, just keep trying. You will succeed as many of my patients have.

21

Exercise

*"Those who think they have no time for
bodily exercise will sooner or later have to
find time for illness."*

*— Edward Stanley (1779 – 1849)
14th Earl of Derby*

Exercise, as you get older, is less appealing and many are unable to do the things they did in their youth. Due to pain or injury, many people cannot do high intensity sports like aerobics, weight training, or basketball.

Everything in moderation

The exercise you do does not have to be strenuous. It doesn't matter what you do as long as you do something. Moderate exercise builds muscle, increases stamina, and produces a host of hormones that make you feel better and improve health. Swimming and biking are two excellent not-so-intense activities that tend to be injury free and can be done your whole life. Gardening and walking are also great way to get your body moving. Make it a habit to walk after dinner or ride a bike daily. You will feel the benefit.

Build up your heart's reserve capacity

Reserve capacity is the heart's ability to pump blood at a moment's notice. Lack of reserve capacity has led to many a heart attack. How many heart attack stories have you heard about someone who, after a period of inactivity, suddenly has to push someone's car, or decides to recapture their youth and play a pickup basketball game? Probably a few. It's because they have little or no reserve capacity.

Always start slow and build up. Do not start *any* exercise program without first consulting your doctor.

The best way to rev up your reserve capacity is with **interval training**. Interval training causes your body to not store calories as fat because it thinks you need it for short bursts of exercise. Ever wonder why tigers look so lean? They lie around most of the day but run in short intervals at full speed to catch their prey.

Determining your workout intensity

To determine how hard or what intensity to work out at:

1. Subtract your age from 220. For example, if you are 53 years old:

    220 (maximum heart rate) - 53 = 167 bpm (beats per minute)

2. Determine your resting heart rate. To do this, rest your forefinger on your wrist and check your pulse at the wrist for six seconds. Multiply the heartbeats by 10.

You want to work out at 75 of 85 percent of that rate. So, for the 53-year-old, that would mean she would want to keep her heart rate between 125 and 142 bpm. Now, this is a little hard to do. Even machines with heart rate monitors do not adjust quickly and accurately enough to let you know where you are at with interval training methods. Some intervals are just 30 seconds and the readings on most machines do not calibrate fast enough. Here's a solution: look at the intensity level of your body's reaction to exercise, where:

Level 1   =   Barely moving
Level 10 =   Running at a full sprint
Level 5   =   Halfway in between

Experiment and you'll get used to the machine you are on and you'll begin to know what levels on the machine correspond to your level of exercise.

For example, on the elliptical training machine at my gym level 12 equals a speed of 7.5 RPM, which translates into level 5 in intensity for me. That's about half as fast as I can go. When I get up to 12 to 13 RPM at level 12, I'm running as fast as I can, or a level 9 in intensity. It takes a little experimenting but you will get the hang of it. It's a general rule, but you will know when you are going all out or at half speed after a few workouts.

Three programs

Just as there is more than one way to skin a cat, there is more than one way to do interval training. I've designed three interval training programs that will increase your reserve capacity and get your body into sugar-burning mode. The programs are similar but differ in duration and intensity.

These training programs are great time savers, keep you interested and, best of all, increase your reserve capacity.

The main differences in the programs are the levels of intensity, duration of intensity, and duration of the rest periods. Also, some rest periods are done at higher levels. Sometimes the rest period is a walking level and sometimes it is a Level 4 intensity.

In one program you are running at high intensity for 1½ minutes and then rest or recovery mode is for 3 minutes; in another the high intensity is for 30 seconds and the lower recovery intensity is for a shorter period of 1½ minutes.

Any long-term exercise program must have variety or most of us get bored and do not stick to it. I recommend mastering each program and then alternating them three to four times a week is at a minimum. They can also be done daily. I recommend doing a long (45 minutes to 1 hour) low intensity aerobic session once a week or every other week to prevent boredom.

Beginner program

You can run in the park with a good watch or timing device or use a treadmill or any one of the many elliptical machines at the local gym to do the programs.

The Beginner program consists of:
1. Warm up for 1 minute at level 3.

2. Interval 1:

    Exercise for 1 minute at level 5
    Rest one minute a level 3

3. Interval 2:

    Exercise for 1 minute at level 6
    Rest for one minute a level 3

4. Interval 3:

    Exercise for 1 minute at level 7
    Rest for one minute a level 4

5. Interval 4:

Exercise for I minute at level 8

Rest for one minute a level 3

6. Interval 5:

Exercise for 30 seconds at level 9

Recovery at level 3 for 2 minutes

This program takes 12 minutes to complete.

Intermediate program

The Intermediate program consists of eight sprints of 30 seconds with 1½-minute rest (recovery) periods as follows:

1. Warm up for 2 minutes at Level 3.

2. Intervals 1 through 8 (repeat 8 times):

Sprint at level 9 for 30 seconds
Slow to level 3 for 1½ minutes

3. Cool down for 2 minutes.

This program takes 20 minutes to complete.

Advanced program

The Advanced program consists of:

1. Warm up for 2 minutes at level 3.

2. Intervals 1 through 4 (repeat 4 times):

Sprint at level 6 for 2 minutes
Recovery at level 3 for 3 minutes

Increase the middle two intervals to level 7 or 8 if you can handle it.

This program takes 22 minutes to complete.

Tracking your progress

To track your progress take your pulse when you are finished exercising and again after two minutes of complete rest. Your pulse should drop by fifty points. If you stop your interval training and your pulse is 142, for example, it should go down to 92 after two minutes rest. It could drop as many as 70 points when you get in really good shape, but anything approaching a 50 point drop after the two minute mark is a good sign of improving cardiac muscle health.

Improving your cardiac health by increasing your reserve capacity is very important. Over exercising with long periods of aerobics can actually stress the body and increase your risk of heart attack. That is counterproductive. Interval training is short and takes only 3 to 4 sessions a week for maximum benefit. Do your heart a favor and start today.

Exercise, diet, and vitamins: a three-pronged attack

You've heard it before and I'm saying it again:
- Eat healthfully
- Exercise
- Take a full spectrum supplement

This three-pronged attack is the best natural prevention and treatment for heart disease you'll find. It has worked for thousands of my patients and it will work for you, too.

Good luck.

22

Conclusion

Threehe bible says in the book of Proverbs 18:17, "The first to present his case seems right until another comes forward to question him." The holistic side is drowned out by the media, drug, and governmental machine. This book is an attempt to tell the other side.

Settling for the paltry results of the medical model that helps a fraction of the patients while they tout reductions of thirty to forty percent under the guise of relative risk reduction is a failed model. How is it possible that a drug would cost 700 million to produce and have such miserable results and such severe side effects?

For example, Avandia has been on the market for close to twenty years and is now under scrutiny for increased heart attack risk for diabetics who take it.

Drug companies continue to produce compounds that are toxic to the body and work by blocking enzyme functions or poisoning metabolic pathways, which is never a good idea. This model always leads to serious consequences in the long run.

My model has always been, as a natural practitioner, to correct the underlying cause of disease whether it's diet, faulty nutrition, or environmental factors first—and then only toxic drugs and surgery when absolutely necessary.

Giving the most up to date information to the public is an important endeavor. I have researched thousands of articles for hundreds of hours to find out the truth.

Wisdom is the proper application of knowledge and I have strived to not only provide information based on current research, but by my own results with over 10,000 patients in thirty years of clinical practice.

Ideal supplement formula ingredients

- Ascorbyl Palmitate
- Biotin (Vit. B-7)
- Calcium Ascorbate
- Calcium (Citrate)
- Chromium (Polynicotinate)
- Citrus Bioflavonoids
- Coenzyme Q-10
- Copper Oxide
- Folic Acid
- Glucosamine Sulfate
- Grape Seed Extract
- Inositol
- L-Proline
- L-Arginine
- L-Cysteine
- L-Lysine Hcl
- L-Carnitine (Tartrate)
- Lutein
- Magnesium Ascorbate
- Magnesium Glycinate,
- Molybdenum Glycinate,
- Niacin (Vit. B-3)
- Niacinamide
- Pantothenic Acid (Vit. B-5) (D-Cal Panto)
- Potassium (Chloride)
- Pycnogenol
- Riboflavin (Vit. B-2)

- Selenium (L-Selenomethionine)
- Thiamine Mononitrate (Vit. B1),
- Trace Minerals
- Vitamin A (Beta Carotene)
- Vitamin B-6 (Pyridoxine Hcl)
- Vitamin B-12 (Cyanocobalamin)
- Vitamin C (Ascorbic Acid)
- Vitamin D-3 (Cholecalciferol)
- Vitamin E (D-Alpha Toco Succinate)
- Zinc Oxide

Of course there are beneficial nutrients for heart health like niacin and fish oils high in omega-3 fatty acids. However, niacin requires special instructions and fish oil can actually be dangerous if not taken in the right form and with the proper co factors.

I have two special reports at www.heartlifenews.com to guide you through this process. But for an essential formula that is foundational to optimum health the above nutrients are critical.

From over forty heart health supplements on the market I have examined only HeartLifePlus by Natures Window has everything in correct dose and amount. Many formulas lack an amino acid blend or have an incorrect blend so you don't get the benefits of say arginine that stops heart attacks and lowers blood pressure or the collagen building benefits of lysine and proline.

Many times formulas don't have the right cofactors like co-enzyme Q-10, which requires a seventeen step process needing multiple b vitamins and minerals. Others don't have the four types of vitamin C or are missing antioxidants like pycnogenol and bioflavonoids and other to factors.

Synergism (where adding nutrients increases their effectiveness) is the most important concept and is woefully absent. It is critical to have all the nutrients in the correct dose and form for maximum health maintenance.

We are all in this boat together. It is important to do something every day for heart health, whether it's the diet, exercise or the supplements.

Stop waiting to become the next casualty. Sign up for my newsletter at drdanpilgreen.com and get weekly updates on heart health from current research around the world. Change starts in the mind and reading this book is a great start to better health. Congratulations. My hope and prayer is for your good health and a fulfilling and long life.

About the Author

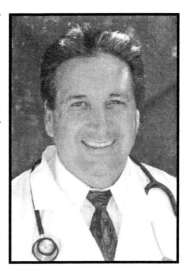

T his book is the result of the journey of an idealistic young doctor who wanted to treat all health conditions, but became disenchanted by the lack of success in areas where conventional methods just didn't work.

Dr. Dan Pilgreen, D.C. practiced holistic medicine as director of the California Chiropractic Clinic in Los Angeles for 23 years, is a board certified Chiropractic Internist and was on the post-graduate faculty of Cleveland Chiropractic College. He graduated as one of the youngest Doctors of Chiropractic in California in 1981 from the Southern California University of Health Sciences and has treated over 10,000 patients, many of whom had heart disease, high blood pressure, and high cholesterol, as well as the usual neck and back pain seen by most chiropractors.

When as a young man he was injured in a serious car accident that left him unable to walk, the medical profession failed to help him regain his ability to walk. He sought chiropractic care, which restored his health, and so inspired him that he dedicated himself to chiropractic medicine to help others.

After Dr. Pilgreen's father died of a heart attack and his mother, a fellow doctor, and even his tennis coach suffered heart attacks as well, he retired from practice to devote himself to researching the true cause of heart disease.

His research spanned six years, including reading over three thousand articles and journals and spending hundreds of hours in postgraduate courses to find the answer.

He uncovered the chiropractic and medical professions' lack of success and outright corruption and the drug companies' ineffectiveness at offering health solutions.

Finally, He discovered an all-natural protocol to prevent heart attacks and the related conditions of high blood pressure, high cholesterol, and diabetes. His effective solution to treat these and many other conditions involves a unique combination the proper nutrition, diet, and exercise.

Dr. Pilgreen then hosted a successful radio program on KRLA 870 AM in Los Angeles discussing the natural treatment of disease for three years.

In this book, he defies medical/pharmaceutical convention and tells the honest truth about the importance of nutrition.

This is truly a breakthrough from a holistic doctor who has worked in the trenches with thousands of patients to get them off drugs and back to health—naturally and without drugs or surgery.

Dr. Pilgreen lives in Los Angeles with his wife and two children. In his leisure hours he plays golf, enjoys cooking organic food, and seeks out new natural cures.

*You reach him at **drdan@drdanpilgreen.com**.*

Resources

Cambell, Colin T. Phd. and Thomas Cambell II. *The China Study: Startling Implications for Diet, Weight Loss and Long-Term Health*, Benbella Books, 2005.

DeFelice, Stephen M.D., *The Carnitine Defense.*, St. Martins Press, 1999.

Fried, Robert Ph.D. and Woodson C, Merrill, M.D. *The Arginine Solution*, Warner Books, 1999.

Hickey, Steve PhD. and Andrew W. Saul Ph,D *Vitamin C: The Real Story.* Basic Health Publications, Inc., 2008.

Houston, Mark M.D., *What your Doctor May Not Tell You About Hypertension*, Hachette Book Group, 2003.

Kaufman, Joel PhD. *Malignant Medical Myths*, West Conshohocken, Infinity Publishing, 2006.

McGee, Charles T. M.D. *Heart Frauds: Uncovering the Biggest Health Scam In History*, Piccadilly Books Ltd., 2007.

Mindell, Earl and Virginia Hopkins, *Prescription Alternatives*, 2nd ed., Keats Publishing, 1999.

Murry, Michael N.D. *Encyclopedia of Nutritional Supplements*, Prima Publishing, 1996.

Niacin report, www.natureswindow.net.

Omega three report, www.natureswindow.net.

Orey, Cal, *The Healing Powers of Olive Oil: A Complete Guide to Nature's Liquid Gold*, Kensington Books, 2009.

Pelton, Ross and James B. LaValle, *The Nutritional Cost of Prescription Drugs*, Morton Publishing Company, 2000.

Pelton, Ross, *Drug Induced Nutrient Depletion Handbook*, Lexi-Comp, Inc., 1999.

PubMed, a website paid by you and run by the government. Here you can find many journals from the U.S. and around the world, such as the Journal of the American Medical Association, British Medical Journal, New England Journal of Medicine.

Ravnskov, Uffe M.D., PhD, *The Cholesterol Myths: Exposing the fallacy that saturated fat and cholesterol cause heart disease*, New Trends Publishing, 2000.

Stone, Irwin. *The Healing Factor*, Grosset & Dunlap, 1972.

Supplement Resources

Centrum: A multi-vitamin that is inadequate based on current scientific research, but will do in a pinch.

HeartLifePlus: The only formula on the market with everything I mention in the book in the right form and dose. http://www.heartlifeplus.com 1-800-600-3099

Index

Your Heart May Be A Ticking Time Bomb!

References

I always try to be like the Bereans, mentioned in book of Acts (17:11), who never believed anything that was preached unless it could be validated by scripture. You should do the same and check the studies and articles for yourself.

To help you, I have attempted to standardize the format of these references and have, where possible, included the name, date, issue, volume, and whatever else might help you find the resource.

[1] Time Magazine, April 28, 2003

[2] "44% of Heart Bypass Surgery is Unneeded," New York Times, Health Section, July 22, 1988.

[3] Open-Heart Surgery Statistics from American Heart Association website. http://www.americanheart.org/presenter.jhtml?identifier=4674 (Accessed February 25, 2009)

[4] M. L. Murphy, et. al. "Treatment of Chronic stable Angina: A preliminary report of survival data of the Randomized Veterans Administration cooperative study." *New England Journal of Medicine* 297, no. 12 (September 22, 1977): 621-627.

[5] Maugh, Thomas H. II "Drug treatment nearly as good as bypass surgery for many patients with severe heart disease." Los Angeles Times (April 4th, 2011).

[6] Brink, Susan. *Extra Car, extra life or extra cost?* Sunday March 12, 2006 L.A. Times

[7] Bangalore, Sripal, MD, MHA, Sabrina Sawhney, MD and Franz H. Messerli, MD. "Relation of Beta-Blocker– Induced Heart Rate Lowering and Cardioprotection in Hypertension." *Journal of American College of Cardiology* vol. 52, issue 18, (October 28, 2008):1482-1489.

[8] Ibid. "44% of Heart Bypass Surgery is Unneeded."

[9] McKeown, L. A., Reviewed by Dr. Tonja Wynn Hampton, "Common Blood Pressure Drug May Not Be So Useful for Heart." WebMD Medical News. http://www.webmd.com/news/20001207/blood-pressure-drug-may-help-heart. (Accessed November 22, 2008).

[10] Pahor, Marco MD et al. "Health outcomes associated with calcium antagonists compared with other first-line antihypertensive therapies: a meta-analysis of randomized controlled trials." The Lancet 356, no. 9246 (December 9, 2000):1949 – 1954.

[11] Lazarou, Jason MSc; Bruce H. Pomeranz, MD, PhD; Paul N. Corey, PhD "Incidence of Adverse Drug Reactions in Hospitalized Patients A Meta-analysis of Prospective Studies." *JAMA* (279) no. 15 (April 15, 1998):1200-1205.

[12] Pelton, Ross et al., Drug-Induced Nutrient Depletion Handbook 1999-2000 (Hudson, Ohio: Lexi-Comp, Inc. 1999),378-383

[13] Serruys, Patrick W., M.D., Ph.D., Marie-Claude Morice, M.D., A. Pieter Kappetein, M.D., Ph.D. et. al "Percutaneous Coronary Intervention versus Coronary-Artery Bypass Grafting for Severe Coronary Artery Disease" *New England Journal of Medicine* 360, no. 10 (March 5, 2009): 961-972 .

[14] Sanket S. Dhruva, MD; Lisa A. Bero, PhD; Rita F. Redberg, MD, MSc "Strength of Study Evidence Examined by the FDA in Premarket Approval of Cardiovascular Devices." *JAMA.* 2009;302(24):2679-2685.

[15] Andraws, Richard MD; Jeffrey S. Berger, MD; David L. Brown, MD. "Effects of Antibiotic Therapy on Outcomes of Patients with Coronary Artery Disease: A Meta-analysis of Randomized Controlled Trials." *Journal of the American Medical Association* 293, no. 12 (June 1, 2005):2641-2647.

[16] Bhatt, Deepak L. et al. "Clopidogrel and Aspirin versus Aspirin Alone for the Prevention of Atherothrombotic Events." *New England Journal of Medicine,* 354 no. 18 (April 20, 2006):1706-1717.

[17] Maugh, Thomas H. II "Study Raises Doubt on Anti-Clotting Drug" From the Los Angeles Times (March 13, 2006).

[18] Ibid., Carlson.

[19] Ibid., Europa Study

[20] Ibid., Pahor

[21] Lazarou, Jason MSc; Bruce H. Pomeranz, MD, PhD; Paul N. Corey, PhD "Incidence of Adverse Drug Reactions in Hospitalized Patients: A Meta-analysis of Prospective Studies" *JAMA* 279, no. 15 (April 15, 1998):1200-1205.

[22] Classen, D. C., S. L. Pestotnik, R. S. Evans, J. F. Lloyd and J. P. Burke Department of Clinical Epidemiology, LDS Hospital, Salt Lake City, UT 84143, USA. "Adverse drug events in hospitalized patients. Excess length of stay, extra costs, and attributable mortality." *JAMA* 277 no., 4 (January 22, 1977).

[23] Ibid. Pearson

[24] Abdel-Aziz Mt, Abdou MS, Soliman K, et al. "Effectsd of L-carnitine on blood lipid patterns in diabetic patients." *Natur Rep Int* 1984; 29:1071-79.

[25] Lubec B. Hayn M, Kitzmuller E., et al. "L-arginine reduces lipid peroxidation in patients with diabetes mellitus." *Free Rad Bio Med* 1997;22:335-57.

[26] *1985 New England Journal of Medicine-"Life* Extension", E.I. Schneider.

[27] Merck Manuel pg.939

[28] 1993 New England Journal of Medicine.

[29] 1992 Dr. Charles Hennekens M.D., Harvard Study.

[30] Harvard Study of 11,00 women.

[31] 1993-Annals of the National Academy of Science, J. M. Gaziano.

[32] 1993-Nutrition intervention trails in Linxian China, Journal of the National cancer Institute, W. J. Blot.

[33] Opotowsky, Alexander R., John P. Bilezikian "'Too much vit. A increases hip fracture risk" *American Journal of Medicine* Vol.117, Issue 3, (August 1, 2004):169-174.

[34] Thomas A. Pearson, M.D., Ph.D., F.A.C.C "Premature CAD With Normal LDL Elevation and Elevated Lp(a)" From the program entitled: Implementing Coronary Risk Factor Modification: Why, How, and In Whom. http://www.acc.org/education/online/risks/cad/index.htm (Accessed April 13, 2008)

[35] Urberg M, Benyi J, John R "Hypocholesterolemic effects of nicotinic acid and chromium supplementation" *Journal of Family Practice* 27, no. 6 December, 1998):603-6.

[36] Maebashi M. et al. "Theraputic evaluation of the theraputic effect of biotin on hyperglycemia in patients with non-insulin dependent diabetes mellitus." *J Clin Biochem Nutr* 1993;14:211-16.

[37] Eric B. Rimm, et al. "Folate and Vitamin B6 from Diet and Supplements in Relation to Risk of Coronary Heart Disease Among Women" *JAMA* Vol. 279 No. 5, (February 4, 1998):359-364.

[38] Joyce, B.B. et al. "Homocysteine Levels and the Risk of Osteoporotic Fracture" *New England Journal of Medicine* 350, no. 20 (May 13, 2004):2033-2041.

[39] McLean, Robert R. et al. "Homocysteine as a Predictive Factor for Hip Fracture in Older Persons" *New England Journal of Medicine.* 350 no. 20 (May 13, 2004):2042-2049.

[40] He K, Merchant A, Rimm EB, Rosner BA, Stampfer MJ, Willett WC, Ascherio A. "Folate, vitamin B6, and B12 intakes in relation to risk of stroke among men." *Stroke* 1 no. 35 (January2004):169-74.

[41] Schnyder, G. et al. "Artery narrowing stopped by B vitamin combination" *New England Journal of Medicine.* 2004; 350 (26):2708-10

[42] Hackam DG, Peterson JC, Spence JD. "What level of plasma homocysteine should be treated? Effects of vitamin therapy on progression of carotid atherosclerosis in patients with homocysteine levels above and below 14 micromol/L." *American Journal of Hypertension* 2000 Jan;13 (1 Pt 1):105-10.

[43] Spence JD, Blake C, Landry A, Fenster A. "Measurement of carotid plaque and effect of vitamin therapy for total homocysteine." *Clin Chem Lab Med.* 2003 Nov:41(11):1498-504.

[44] Seshadri, Sudha, M.D., Alexa Beiser, Ph.D., Jacob Selhub, Ph.D., et al. "Plasma Homocysteine as a Risk Factor for Dementia and Alzheimer's Disease" *New England Journal of Medicine* vol. 346, no. 7 (February 14, 2002):476-483.

[45] Ceriello, J Antonio MD et. Al "Long-term glycemic control influences the long-lasting effect of hyperglycemia on endothelial function in type 1 diabetes" *Journal of Clinical Endocrinology & Metabolism* (June 2, 2009).

[46] Willis, C. G. "The Reversibility of Atherosclerosis." *Can Med Assoc J.* 77, no. 2 (July 15, 1957): 106–109.

[47] Frei B, England L, Ames BN. "Ascorbate is an outstanding antioxidant in human blood plasma." *Proc Natl Acad Sci USA.* 1989;86:6377–6381

[48] Carr, A. C., Zhu BZ, Frei B. "Potential antiantherogenic mechanisms of ascorbate (vitamin C) and alphatocopherol (vitamin E)." *Circulation Research* 87, no. 5 (Sept. 1, 2000):349-54.

[49] Drossos, George E. "Is vitamin C superior to diltiazem for radial artery vasodilation in patients awaiting coronary artery bypass grafting?" *J Thorac Cardiovasc Surg* 2003;125:330.

[50] Stamler, R. et al. "Nutritional therapy for high blood pressure Final report of a four-year randomized controlled trial--the Hypertension Control Program." *JAMA* 257, no. 11 (March 20, 1987).

[51] Mullan, Brian A. "*Lipid* and Protein Metabolism in Type II Diabetes" *Hypertension* 40 (October 21, 2002):804-809.

[52] Kurl S., MD, et al. "Plasma Vitamin C Modifies the Association between Hypertension and Risk of Stroke." *JAMA* 33, no. 6 (June 1,2002):1568.

[53] Gatto, L. M. ,G. K. Hallen, A. J. Brown and S. Samman "Ascorbic Acid induces a favorable lipoprotein profile in women." *Journal of the American College of Nutrition*, Vol 15, Issue 2 (1996):154-158.

[54] Ness, A. R. et al. "Vitamin C status and serum lipids." *European Journal of clinical Nutrition* 11, no. 50 (Nov. 1996):724-729

[55] Stavroula, K et al. "Vitamin C and risk of coronary heart disease in women." Journal of the American College of Cardiology 42 (2003):246-252.

[56] Knekt, Paul "Antioxidant vitamins and coronary heart disease risk: a pooled analysis of 9 cohorts." *American Journal of Clinical Nutrition*, Vol. 80, No. 6 (December 2004):1508-1520.

[57] Enstrom, J.E., Kanim LE, Klein MA "Vitamin C intake and mortality among a sample of the United States population" *Epidemiology* 3, no. 3 (MAY, 1992):194-202.

[58] Losonczy, K. G., TB Harris and RJ Havlik "Vitamin E and vitamin C supplement use and risk of all-cause and coronary heart disease mortality in older persons: the Established Populations for Epidemiologic Studies of the Elderly." *American Journal of Clinical Nutrition*, Vol. 64 (1996):190-196.

[59] Simon, Joel A. MD, MPH; Esther S. Hudes, PhD, MPH "Relationship of Ascorbic Acid to Blood Lead Levels." *JAMA* vol. 281, No.24 (June 23,1999):2289-2293.

[60] Dawson, Earl B. PhD, et al. "The Effect of Ascorbic Acid Supplementation on the Blood Lead Levels of Smokers." *Journal of the American College of Nutrition*, Vol. 18, No. 2, (April, 1999):166-170.

[61] Woodward M, Lowe GD, Rumley A, et al. "Epidemiology of coagulation factors, inhibitors and activation markers: the third Glasco MONICA survey." *Br J Haematol* 1997;97:785-97.

[62] Khaw, K. T., Woodhouse P. "Interrelation of vitamin C, infection, hemostatic factors, and cardiovascular disease." *BMJ* 1995;310:1559-63.

[63] Bordia AK. "The effect of vitamin C on blood lipids, fibrinolytic activity and platelet adhesiveness in patients with coronary artery disease." *Atherosclerosis* 1980;35:181-7.

[64] Bordia A, Verma SK. "Effect of vitamin C on platelet adhesiveness and platelet aggregation in coronary artery disease patients." *Clin Cardiol* 1985;8:552-4.

[65] Willis, C. G. "The Reversibility of Atherosclerosis." *Can Med Assoc J.* 77, no. 2 (July 15, 1957): 106-109.

[66] Journal of Applied Nutrition (1996) 48: 68-78.

[67] The American Journal of Clinical Nutrition, 2008.

[68] Grant WB, Garland CF, Gorham ED. "An estimate of cancer mortality rate reductions in Europe and the US with 1,000 IU of oral vitamin D per day." *Recent Results Cancer Res.* 2007;174:225-34. http://www.ncbi.nlm.nih.gov/pubmed/17302200 (Accessed Dec. 5, 2008)

[69] Makishima, Makoto, Timothy T. Lu, Wen Xie "Vitamin D Receptor As an Intestinal Bile Acid Sensor." *Science* Vol. 296. no. 5571 (May 17 2002): 1313 – 1316.

[70] Ibid, Skinner

[71] Tenkanen L, Syvala H, Lumme S. et al. "Interaction of factors related to the metabolic syndrome and vitamin D on risk of prostate cancer." *Cancer Epidemiol Biomarkers Prev.* 16, no. 2 (Feb. 2007):302-7.

[72] Shoji T, Nishizawa Y. Osaka City University Graduate School of Medicine, Depanartment of Metabolism, Endocrinology and Molecular Medicine. "Effects of vitamin D on the cardiovascular system" *Clin Calcium.* 2006 Jul;16 (7):1107-14.

[73] Zittermann A, Schleithoff SS, Tenderich G, Berthold HK, Korfer R, Stehle P. Department of Nutrition Science, University of Bonn, Germany "Low vitamin D status: a contributing factor in the pathogenesis of congestive heart failure?" *J Am Coll Cardiol.* 41 no. 1(Jan. 1, 2003):105-12.

[74] Hein G, Oelzner P. "Vitamin D metabolites in rheumatoid arthritis: findings--hypotheses— consequences." *Z Rheumatol.* 2000; 59 Suppl 1:28-32.

[75] Timms PM, Mannan N, Hitman GA et al. "Circulating MMP9, vitamin D and variation in the TIMP-1 response with VDR genotype: mechanisms for inflammatory damage in chronic disorders?" *QJM (Monthly Journal of the Association of Physicians)* 2002 Dec; 95 (12):787-96.

[76] Lee, I-Min et al. "Vitamin E in the Primary Prevention of cardiovascular Disease and Cancer The Women's Health Study: A Randomized Controlled Trial" *JAMA* vol. 294 no. 1, (July 6, 2005):56-65.

[77] Heinonen, Olli P., Demetrius Albanes "Vitamin E Reduces Prostate Cancer Rates in Finnish Trial: U.S. Considers Follow-up." *Journal of the National Cancer Institute* Vol. 90 no. 5 (1998):416-417.

Your Heart May Be A Ticking Time Bomb!

[78] Stephens NG; Parsons A; Schofield PM; Kelly F; Cheeseman K; Mitchinson MJ "Randomised controlled trial of vitamin E in patients with coronary disease: Cambridge Heart Antioxidant Study (CHAOS)." *Lancet,* 347(9004):781-6 1996 Mar 23.

[79] Stampfer Meir J., Charles H. Hennekens, JoAnn E. Manson, et al. "Vitamin E Consumption and the Risk of Coronary Disease in Women." *New England Journal of Medicine* vol. 20 no. 328 (May 20, 1993):1444-1449.

[80] Rimm, Eric B., Meir J. Stampfer, Alberto Ascherio, et al. "Vitamin E consumption and risk of coronary artery disease" *New England Journal of Medicine* vol. 328, no. 20 (May 20, 1993):1450-1456.

[81] Devaraj, Sridevi "Vitamin E Lowers C-Reactive Protein and IL-6" *Free Radical Biology & Medicine*- Official Journal of the Society for Free Radical Biology and Medicine. October 23, 2000.

[82] Wright, Margaret E, Karla A Lawson, Stephanie J Weinstein, et al. "Higher baseline serum concentrations of vitamin E are associated with lower total and cause-specific mortality in the Alpha-Tocopherol, Beta-Carotene Cancer Prevention Study1,2,3." *American Journal of Clinical Nutrition,* Vol. 84, No. 5, (November 2006):1200-1207.

[83] Archives of Neurology July 2002;59:1125-1132.

[84] Ford, Earl S. and Anne Sowell "In a study done by the Serun α-Tochopherol Status in the United States Population: Findings from The Third National Health and Nutrition Examination Survey" The Johns Hopkins University School of Hygiene and Public Health American *Journal of Epidemiology* Vol. 150, No. 3(1999): 290-300.

[85] Plotnick GD, Corretti MC, Vogel RA. "Effect of antioxidant vitamins on the transient impairment of endothelium-dependent brachial artery vasoactivity following a single high-fat meal." *JAMA* 1997;278:1682-6.

[86] Zavaroni, I et al. "Risk factors for coronary artery disease in healthy persons with hyperinsulinemia and normal glucose tolerance." *New England Journal of Medicine* vol. 320 no. 11 (March 16, 1998):702-706.

[87] Press RI, Geller J, Evans GW. "The effect of chromium picolinate on serum cholesterol and apolipoprotein fractions in human subjects." *West J Med.* 1990 Jan;152(1):41-5.

[88] J Urberg M, Benyi J, John R. "Hypocholesterolemic effects of nicotinic acid and chromium supplementation." *Fam Pract.* 1988 Dec;27(6):603-6.

[89] Crawford V, Scheckenbach R, Preuss HG. "Effects of niacin-bound chromium supplementation on body composition in overweight African-American women." *Diabetes Obes Metab.* 1999 Nov;1(6):331-7.

[90] *American Journal of Physiology* 709 (1065):433-7.

[91] Proceedings of the 5th International Symposium on Atherosclerosis Huston, TX 1979.

[92] American Journal of Clinical Nutrition 34(1991):2670-8.

[93] Preuss HG, Wallerstedt D, Talpur N, et al. "Effects of niacin-bound chromium and grape seed proanthocyanidin extract on the lipid profile of hypercholesterolemic subjects: a pilot study." *J Med.* 2000;31(5-6):227-46.

[94] Rabinovitz H, Friedensohn A, Leibovitz A, Gabay G, Rocas C, Habot B. "Effect of chromium supplementation on blood glucose and lipid levels in type 2 diabetes mellitus elderly patients." *Int J Vitam Nutr Res.* 2004 May;74(3):178-82.

[95] Miranda ER, Dey CS. "Effect of chromium and zinc on insulin signaling in skeletal muscle cells." *Biol Trace Elem Res.* 2004 Oct;101(1):19-36.

[96] Age-Related Eye Disease Study Research Group "A Randomized, Placebo-Controlled, Clinical Trial of High-Dose Supplementation with Vitamins C and E, Beta Carotene, and Zinc for Age-Related Macular Degeneration and Vision Loss" AREDS Report No. 8 *Arch Ophthalmol.* 119, 10 (October, 2001):1417-1436.

[97] Ravaglia, Giovanni, Paola Forti, Fabiola Maioli et al. "Blood Micronutrient and Thyroid Hormone Concentrations in the Oldest-Old." *The Journal of Clinical Endocrinology & Metabolism* Vol. 85, No. 6 (June 2000):2260-5.

[98] Ruz, M. et al. "Single and multiple selenium-zinc-iodine deficiencies affect rat thyroid metabolism and ultra structure." *Journal Nutrition* 129, 1 (January 1999):174-80.

[99] Peretz A, et al. *Semin Arthritis Rheum* vol. 20 no. 5 (Apr 1991):305-316.

[100] Clark, Larry C., MPH, PhD; Gerald F. Combs, Jr, PhD et al. "Effects of Selenium Supplementation for Cancer Prevention in Patients With Carcinoma of the Skin A Randomized Controlled Trial." *JAMA* 1996;276(24):1957-1963.

[101] Klaus K.A. Witte, Nikolay P. Nikitin, Anita C. Parker et al. "The effect of micronutrient supplementation on quality-of-life and left ventricular function in elderly patients with chronic heart failure." *European Heart Journal* 26, no 21(Nov. 1, 2005): 2238-2244.

[102] Leslie M Klevay "Extra dietary copper inhibits LDL oxidation." *American Journal of Clinical Nutrition*, Vol. 76, No. 3, (September 2002): 687-688.

[103] Rock E, Mazur A, O'Connor JM, Bonham MP, Rayssiguier Y, Strain JJ. "The effect of copper supplementation on red blood cell oxidizability and plasma antioxidants in middle-aged healthy volunteers." *Free Radic Biol Med* 2000;28:324–9.

[104] Peter A. McCullough, et al., "Confirmation of a heart failure epidemic: findings from the Resource Utilization Among Congestive Heart Failure (REACH) study." *J Am Coll Cardiol.* 2002; 39:60-69.

[105] *Current Therapeutic Research* Vol. 51 (1992):668-672.

[106] Cho KJ, Yun CH, Packer L, Chung AS. "Inhibition mechanisms of bioflavonoids extracted from the bark of Pinus maritima on the expression of proinflammatory cytokines." *Ann N Y Acad Sci.* 2001 Apr;928:141-56.

[107] Li WG, Zhang XY, Wu YJ, Tian X. "Anti-inflammatory effect and mechanism of proanthocyanidins from grape seeds." *Acta Pharmacol Sin.* 2001 Dec;22(12):1117-20.

[108] Cesarone MR, Belcaro G, Stuard S, Schönlau F, et al. "Kidney flow and function in hypertension: protective effects of pycnogenol in hypertensive participants--a controlled study." *J Cardiovasc Pharmacol Ther.* 2010 Mar;15(1):41-6. Epub 2010 Jan 22.

[109] Hertog, M.G.L, E.J.M Feskens , D Kromhout PhD et al. "Dietary antioxidant flavonoids and risk of coronary heart disease: the Zutphen Elderly Study." *Lancet*, Volume 342, Issue 8878(23 October 1993):1007 – 1011.

[110] Steigerwalt R, Belcaro G, Cesarone MR et al. "Pycnogenol improves microcirculation, retinal edema, and visual acuity in early diabetic retinopathy." *J Ocul Pharmacol Ther.* 2009 Dec;25(6):537-40.

[111] Rohdewald P. "A review of the French maritime pine bark extract (Pycnogenol), a herbal medication with a diverse clinical pharmacology." *Int J Clin Pharmacol Ther.* 2002 Apr;40(4):158-68.

[112] Ibid

[113] Deters A, Petereit F, Schmidgall J, Hensel A. "N-Acetyl-D-glucosamine oligosaccharides induce mucin secretion from colonic tissue and induce differentiation of human keratinocytes." *J Pharm Pharmacol.* 2008 Feb;60(2):197-204.

[114] Ma L, Lin XM. "Effects of lutein and zeaxanthin on aspects of eye health." *J Sci Food Agric.* 2010 Jan 15;90(1):2-12.

[115] Izumi-Nagai K, Nagai N, Ohgami K "Macular pigment lutein is antiinflammatory in preventing choroidal neovascularization." *Arterioscler Thromb Vasc Biol.* 2007 Dec;27(12):2555-62.

[116] Arnal E, Miranda M, Almansa I, "Lutein prevents cataract development and progression in diabetic rats." *Graefes Arch Clin Exp Ophthalmol.* 2009 Jan;247(1):115-20.

Your Heart May Be A Ticking Time Bomb!

[117] "Clinical trial of lutein in patients with retinitis pigmentosa receiving vitamin A" *Arch Ophthalmol.* 2010 Apr;128(4):403-11.

[118] Izumi-Nagai K, Nagai N, Ohgami K "Macular pigment lutein is anti-inflammatory in preventing choroidal neovascularization." *Arterioscler Thromb Vasc Biol.* 2007 Dec;27(12):2555-62.

[119] 1994 Journal of Nutrition, no.124 pp. 1060-106.

[120] 1996 Journal of the American Medical Association no. 272, pp 1016-1022.

[121] Heiner C. Bucher; Gordon H. Guyatt; Richard J. Cook et al. "Effect of Calcium Supplementation on Pregnancy-Induced Hypertension and Preeclampsia: A Meta-analysis of Randomized Controlled Trials." JAMA. 1996;275(14):1113-1117.

[122] Griffith, Lauren E.,Gordon H. Guyatt, Richard J. Cook, et al. "The influence of dietary and nondietary calcium supplementation on blood pressure" Am J Hypertens (1999) 12:84-92.

[123] Science,1980 208 :198-200.

[124] 1992 Journal of the American Medical Association, 268:2395-2402.

[125] 1993 American Journal of Hypertension, 6:41-45.

[126] JC Witteman, et al. "Reduction of blood pressure with oral magnesium supplementation in women with mild to moderate hypertension." American Journal of Clinical Nutrition, 1994 Vol 60,p 129-135.

[127] Champagne, Catherine M.PhD,RD,LDN,FADA "Magnesium in Hypertension, Cardiovascular Disease, Metabolic Syndrome, and Other Conditions:A Review of Nutrition" in Clinical Practice Vol.23,No. 2,(2008):142-151.

[128] Whelton, P K et al. "Potassium in preventing and treating high blood pressure." Seminars in Nephrology 1999;19:494-499.

[129] BARRI, YOUSRI M.; WINGO, CHARLES S. "The Effects of Potassium Depletion and Supplementation on Blood Pressure: A Clinical Review." American Journal of the Medical Sciences. (July 1997) 314(1):37-40.

[130] Sacks, Frank M. "Effect on Blood Pressure of Potassium, Calcium, and Magnesium in Women With Low Habitual Intake." Hypertension 1998;31:131

[131] 1990 "Biological and Clinical Relevance of Trace Elements" Arztl Lab 36:284-287

[132] 1991 Cancer Causes and Controls, 427-442, Stienmetz.

[133] U.S. Department of Health and Human Services National Institutes of Health National Institute on Aging "Centenarians in the United States" P23199RV Current Population Reports Published July 1999.

[134] Ross L. Prentice, PhD; Bette Caan, DrPH et. Al. "Low-Fat Dietary Pattern and Risk of Invasive Breast Cancer" *JAMA* vol. 295 No. 6 (Feb. 8, 2006);629-642; Shirley A. A. Beresford, PhD; Karen C. Johnson, et al. "Low-Fat Dietary Pattern and Risk of Colorectal Cancer" *JAMA* vol. 295 No. 6 (Feb. 8, 2006);64329-654; Barbara V. Howard, PhD; Linda Van Horn, PhD, et. Al. "Low-Fat Dietary Pattern and Risk of Cardiovascular Disease" *JAMA* vol. 95 No. 6 (Feb. 8, 2006); 655-666.

[135] Scarmeas, N, Stern Y, Mayeux R, et. al. "Mediterranean diet and mild cognitive impairment" Archives of Neurology 2009 Feb; 66(2);216-25.

[136] Lorgeril, Michel de, Patricia Salen, Jean-Louis Martin, Isabelle Monjaud, Jacques Delaye, and Nicole Mamelle "Mediterranean Diet, Traditional Risk Factors, and the Rate of Cardiovascular Complications After Myocardial Infarction : Final Report of the Lyon Diet Heart Study" Circulation Vol. 99, Issue 6 (February 16, 1999):779-785.

[137] Ferrara, L.A., et al. "Olive oil and reduced need for antihypertensive medication" Archives of Internal Medicine 2000; 160:837-842.